D1167602

# The StressProof Life

---

## The Secret to Health, Wealth, and Happiness

## Amir A. Rashidian, D.C.

www.midatlantic
clinic.com

Health@DrRashidian.com

The StressProof Life
The Secret to Health, Wealth, and Happiness
ISBN: 978-0-9963001-3-1
Author: Amir A. Rashidian, D.C.

1st Printing, February 2016
2nd Printing, January 2017
Printed in the United States of America

# Dedication

This book is dedicated to my amazing wife, Brandi, who one day said, "You have eight months before the baby is born. That should be plenty of time for you to finish your book." Today, that baby is 5 years old. Thank you for your patience, honey. I love you.

This book is also dedicated to my two sons, Navid and Ramin. Every day I am inspired by the strength and courage with which you face every challenge. I am humbled by the incredible kindness that you both possess in your hearts. You are each a gift from God and I am so privileged and honored to be your dad. I love you.

Last but not least, this book is dedicated to my patients. Your trust and loyalty are invaluable and I am so incredibly grateful to be a part of your lives. Over the past fifteen years you have taught me how to be a true doctor and I hope to continue this incredible journey with you. I know that together we can StressProof our lives and build a healthier next generation. I honor you.

# Acknowledgments

First and foremost, I would like to acknowledge Ms. Jana Warren. Thank you for putting in so much of your heart as well as your personal time to read and edit this book. You are so giving and caring, and this book would not have been completed without your help. I am indebted to you.

To Homa joon and Homeira joon, thank you so much for all of your love and support throughout this process. You have been a tremendous help and the boys are so incredibly blessed to have you in their lives.

To Kadi and Chad Englehart, thank you for all your help and encouragement over the past 8 months. You are both so intelligent and your "fingerprints" are all over this book. Also, you have had such a great positive impact on the practice and for that too, I am grateful.

To Dr. Andrew J. Laflin, thank you for all your support and accountability in helping me finish this book. Thank you also for being my chiropractor and keeping me healthy. God has gifted you with a great heart and great hands and I am grateful to have benefited from both.

To Katelyn Laflin, thank you for being so supportive of your husband, Dr. Andrew, while he put in long hours at the office. Thank you also, for being available and so helpful at the office every time we needed you.

Thank you to all past and present employees of the Mid-Atlantic Chiropractic Center.

Dr. Kenneth J. Williams, you are my brother in every sense of the word. Every time I felt stuck while writing this book, your advice helped me to get back on track. Thank you so much, for so many things, too numerous to list. Thanks also to the lovely Kiri, and my nephews Luke, Cole, and Quin.

Steve Hankins, your friendship means the world to me. I admire your character and faith-filled approach to life and business. I feel empowered by your example. Thank you for always encouraging me. Thanks also to Dr. Carole for being so fantastic. To Ryan and Brandon, thank you for being such great role models for Navid and Ramin.

To Mike and Chrissy Mayhew, thank you so much for persistently encouraging me to write this book and spread my message. I have learned so much from our friendship and we have definitely had great fun along the way. To Andy Mayhew, you are a hero to my boys and I am thankful to have been able to watch you grow up.

Ed Robinson, thank you for your time, your advice, and your friendship over the past 8 years. If it weren't for you, I would still be working on this book. Thank you!

To my Vistage Brothers and Sisters, past and present members, meeting regularly with you was instrumental in finishing this book. I hope that I can give back to you some of what I have received in support and advice.

To Dr. Jim Flood, your guidance and encouragement have helped me through some difficult times and I'm so thankful to have you as a mentor.

Dr. Danny Drubin, thank you for your mentorship. You are a role model to me. Thank you also for the occasional and well-deserved butt-kicking.

Dr. Patrick Gentempo, I am honored to know you. Thank you for bringing the Ultimate Achievers together. That has been one of the most influential aspects of my professional life.

Dr. Kevin Watson, thank you so much for sharing your story with me and allowing me to use it to inspire others.

To Bruce Johnson, my coach and my friend, thank you for your friendship and the incredible wisdom you have shared with me over the past 19 years.

To Bo Eason, I appreciate all your help and encouragement. You are one of the major reasons I was able to write this book.

To Roberto Monaco, I thank you greatly for teaching me how to refine my message and properly communicate with others.

Dr. Christopher Kent, the chiropractic profession and all its patients owe you a debt of gratitude.

A special thank you to my colleagues and fellow chiropractors. You inspire me.

# Table of Contents

# Table of Contents

# Prologue

*At the age of nine, he was staring into the eyes of this young woman who was just told she wouldn't live to see the next day...*

# The StressProof Life

It was a beautiful morning.

Amir Abdolazim, the nine year old boy held his father's hand as they walked through the rural village of small, primitive mud houses nestled near the pure river that ran along a green mountainside. He felt the crisp clean air as it entered his lungs. There was no smog, no power lines, and none of the telephone poles that cluttered his home city of Sari. He saw a shepherd with his flock in the distance, women washing clothes in the river, children playing with sticks and stones. It felt so peaceful there.

It was as if they had gone 200 years back in time.

The tranquil scene was broken by a frantic man screaming something in his native language of Farsi. He was panicked and distraught. Even though young Amir spoke the same language, this man spoke in a dialect that was unfamiliar. Villagers rushed from everywhere to help. The desperate man led his neighbors into his home, the boy and his father followed close behind. The one-room house they entered was rustic but tidy, with pots and pans stacked under a long wooden table, large cushions lay against the wall and an earthen floor was covered by a red hand-woven rug.

But all the boy could see was the groaning woman lying on some blankets in the corner. He felt deep concern for her.

She was obviously pregnant and in a lot of pain. Tears rolled down her cheeks. She screamed in agony and Amir grasped his father's hand tighter. Something didn't feel right about her appearance. No one knew what to do for her. So they waited and watched and suffered with her. Finally, Zahra, the midwife, walked in. She knelt down, examined the woman for a minute or two then stood up. In her native tongue she said, "I'm sorry, the baby is dead, and the mother's time is short. Unless you can get her to a hospital in the next 20 minutes, she will die." With a last look, Zahra walked out the door.

The room was silent except for the pregnant woman's groans. One by one, the villagers left. They knew she would never survive a grueling 2 hour mule ride down the mountain. They shuffled out with their heads low, not making eye contact. A look of horror covered her husband's face as realization of her imminent death dawned and he fell to his knees. He cried in agony, kneeling and holding his arms outstretched toward the sky.

Amir started to cry. He felt pain. It was the first time in his life that an emotion was so strong it felt like physical pain. He felt like he was suffocating. He gasped for air.

His father, Javad, picked him up, held him close, and carried him out of the house. "Amir, my son, there was nothing that could be done. We could not help her. We have to accept that."

He nodded, but he didn't accept it. The image of that woman suffering and slowly dying while her husband sat powerless beside her, was burned into his mind forever. He could not imagine how the emotions of that day would ultimately change the entire course of his life.

With his dad, they made their way down the mountain and got in the car for the three hour drive home.

"Amir, what is it you are thinking about?" asked Javad while driving.

"Baba, I don't want to feel that helpless ever again," the boy stammered, still shaken by the events of the day.

"What do you intend to do about it?"

"I'm going to become a surgeon. I will be the best surgeon in the whole world, and I will carry my bag with me everywhere I go. Baba, I'm going to save lives." With every cell of his nine-year old body and pure determination in his heart, he vowed that he would do whatever it takes to become the world's greatest doctor.

This became his life's purpose.

Ten years later, Amir Abdolazim was a sophomore at The George Washington University in Washington, DC. He was a pre-medical student with stellar grades and every aspect of his life was advancing according to plan; to go to medical school and ultimately save lives. As fate would have it, everything was about to change!

After completing a difficult semester Amir was ready for a much needed rest. He was excited about spending Christmas break at home and seeing his parents who had immigrated to the United States and were now living in Gaithersburg, Maryland. What he experienced as he walked through the door of the small townhouse wasn't the happy and welcoming reception that he expected. His mom and dad didn't rush to the door with outstretched arms and warm embraces. Instead, his dad, Javad, who was wearing a big, thick, white neck brace, walked gingerly toward him. He was obviously heavily medicated and couldn't lift his arms to hug his son. His mother, despite her best efforts couldn't mask the anguish and stress that Javad's injury had caused.

"Hello! Welcome home son! How are you?" asked Javad, as he struggled to smile for his son.

"I'm fine Dad," he replied, but what he really wanted to say was "I can't believe you're in pain again." Javad's condition was a chronic one and seemed to flare up at the most inopportune times. About 10 years prior, he had been involved in several back-to-back car accidents and ever since had suffered from painful episodes, but never this badly.

Amir was disappointed because he wanted to spend time with his dad and enjoy his Christmas break, but Javad was in no condition to socialize.

Javad was in constant pain despite being on strong pain medicine. The excruciating pain started in his neck, shot down his arms, all the way down to his fingertips. His condition had deteriorated so much that he had no strength in his hands. He needed help with the simplest tasks like eating or getting dressed. He couldn't even lie down to go to sleep. He had to sleep in a chair because laying his head back put too much pressure on his neck. So he sat upright, all night in a chair, in the dark, all alone.

As debilitating as the pain was, Javad's emotional stress was even worse. This was because he could no longer do what he loved. He had a passion for writing. He loved to create poems, stories, and jokes. He was an amazing story teller and captivated his audience with his imaginative tales. Bedtime stories with Dad were Amir's favorite memories of his childhood.

Javad also regularly wrote letters to local politicians, senators, and even the president. He enjoyed sharing his ideas on how the president could better do his job. Now he couldn't even hold a pen. He couldn't do what he loved doing the most and he was depressed.

During that Christmas break, Amir took his father to meet with several different doctors. Each doctor they saw referred them to see a different doctor. No one was providing any hope. The two finally ended up at a neurosurgeon's office. "Javad, you needed surgery a long time ago! Why didn't you come to see me sooner?" asked the surgeon not even expecting an answer.

"I'm almost afraid to ask, what kind of surgery?"

"At this point, there isn't much else we can do. The discs in your neck have degenerated and bone spurs are growing into the spinal canal and compressing the spinal cord," said the doctor in a monotone and unemotional voice. He sounded so confident and secure in his opinion that when he said, "surgery is your only option", they believed him. He explained the procedure to them and asked them to call and schedule the surgery.

"Baba, do you realize how invasive this operation is going to be? He said he's going to break and remove the bones in the back of your neck and insert metal rods and screws to fuse your whole neck. You will never turn your head again and you may not regain function of your hands." As Amir was recounting the doctor's graphic description of the surgery, he started to get emotional, and rightfully so, because the doctor had also told them there was a high risk that his dad could die while in surgery because of his age.

Javad was seventy years old, but the recent stresses of his life had caused him to age faster than his peers.

They decided to get a second opinion, hoping for a better prognosis.

The second neurosurgeon said exactly the same thing. As did the third surgeon. "Go and get your affairs in order. We will operate next week", the surgeon ordered nonchalantly.

Disappointed and discouraged, Amir and his father solemnly slid into the cold backseat of the yellow taxi to go home. Amir sat holding the heavy stack of his father's x-rays, MRI's, and medical records. He turned to look at his dad who sat next to him. It broke his heart to see his dad that way. Javad grimaced with every bump that taxi hit because each time, it sent a lightning bolt of pain through his entire body. Looking at his dad at that moment he got the feeling that Javad was tired of living like this, and that he wanted to die.

In that moment, he was emotionally transported back to that village 10 years prior, where he witnessed the young woman die in her husband's arms. He felt the same helplessness that he felt then, except this time he was watching his own father suffer. It was enough to make him second-guess his entire life's plan.

He thought, "Is this the type of news I'll have to give my patients when I'm a surgeon? Will I have to tell them that by operating on them they could lose their life? I don't think I can do that."

Dissecting every possible scenario in his mind he thought, "What if we opt for the operation and he dies? What if we opt for the operation and he isn't any better afterwards? What if we choose not to operate and I watch my dad suffer and slowly die?" The internal dialogue was fueling his emotions and he began to get choked up, his chest felt tight, he struggled to take a full breath, and his eyes filled with tears. He thought he was going to explode. This was exactly how he had felt in that village all those years ago. This feeling is what made him choose to devote his life to becoming a surgeon.

The taxi driver noticed Javad's pain.

"Sir, I see that you're in a lot of pain. I know of this chiropractor just down the street from here. I don't know what he does but I know he helps people like you. Would you like me to take you there?" Despondent, frustrated, and exhausted, with nothing to lose, they agreed.

When they got there, the place seemed to be under construction. They knocked and knocked until a man finally opened the door. He was a calm, relaxed man with streaks of gray in his hair. He introduced himself as Dr. Moretti, the chiropractor, and explained that he was in the middle of building out the suite to move his practice there.

He welcomed them in, walked them past the construction crew putting up dry wall, and offered them tea. Since there was no place to sit, he brought out crates for them to sit on. He also brought with him a light box on which to read the MRI's and x-rays they had brought. As he asked Javad about his condition and how it was affecting his life. He took notes and spent what seemed to be an eternity studying the MRI's and x-rays.

With confidence he finally said, "I can help you. I won't do it by breaking and removing any bones from your spine and I certainly won't insert metal rods and screws into your neck."

This sounded good so far, maybe too good, Amir thought to himself. "What I will do is perform gentle and specific chiropractic adjustments to gradually reduce tension on the spinal cord" Dr. Moretti finished, sensing Amir's skepticism.

"You know, we just met with three of the best neurosurgeons in the country and they all agreed that surgery is the only option. What makes you think you can help my dad?" Amir spoke with a condescending tone. Concerned that Dr. Moretti would be offended, Javad firmly put his hand on Amir's knee to remind him to be respectful.

"I won't lie to you. It's going to be a long, hard, and potentially painful road ahead, but if you don't want surgery, this is your option. It's going to take at least 6 months before you notice a change in your condition and you will need to see me 6 days a week during those first six months. Are you prepared to make that kind of commitment?" Amir was still reluctant but saw a spark of hope in his father. Javad was willing to try anything just to avoid the dangerous surgery, so he agreed.

That same day, after a thorough physical exam, Dr. Moretti gave Javad his very first chiropractic adjustment.

The movement was swift and small, hardly noticeable. But the sound was crisp, loud and clear. Javad smiled, which was rare these days and said, "Wow!" He lay quietly for a moment. "It feels like you just poured cold water on a hot flame. That's exactly what I needed." By the time Javad stood up after his adjustment, all of his excruciating symptoms had returned, but he now had hope that over time his body could heal.

Javad faithfully went to see Dr. Moretti the chiropractor, six days a week for the next six months. After the first month, he didn't personally think he was feeling any better, but everyone around him had noticed that he had stopped getting worse. His condition seemed to have stabilized.

So he kept going.

Six and a half months passed and just as he had done almost every day until then, Javad walked into the reception room of Dr. Moretti's office. The construction had been completed. Comfortable chairs replaced the original primitive crates and a beautiful granite counter separated the room from the receptionist who stood behind it. The office was very busy and there were patients in every seat waiting to be seen by Dr. Moretti.

Javad confidently walked up to the counter, picked up the pen and paused as he held it in his hand. With a big smile on his face and without assistance he wrote his name on the sign-in sheet. To the average person this may seem insignificant but it was the first time in over a year that he had been able to write with a pen. Then he took that pen and held it high over his head as if lifting a trophy. He was celebrating. The patients in the reception area did not understand but they smiled regardless. The receptionist behind the counter, a young woman in her late twenties with auburn hair and large brown eyes, started to cry. Every time Javad had walked into that office she had been the one to write his name for him on the sign-in sheet. When Javad had started to gain some strength in his hands, she would hold his hand for him and try to guide it as he wrote. But each time he attempted, he would drop the pen and he would get frustrated. But on that day and every day after that, Javad was able to perform the task of writing on his own. Once again he could pursue his passion, and guess who started receiving letters from Javad again? Yes, the president and senators.

Javad lived another 18 years after that. At the age of 88, he seemed younger than he was at 70. He woke up early every morning to exercise. Then he would head out the door to visit his friends, most of whom were confined to nursing homes. He was self-sufficient and traveled regularly, both across the country and abroad. He lived a good life, enjoying every moment.

And I, Amir Abdolazim Rashidian, am the boy from this story. I was the 9 year-old boy who Javad took to that village in the foothills of the Elburz Mountain range, the child who witnessed the pregnant woman pass away in the arms of her husband, the one who decided to dedicate the rest of his life to becoming a doctor in order to save lives, the one who is eternally grateful to have been in that particular taxi that important day, and indebted to the chiropractor who gave my father, Javad Rashidian, his life back.

Thanks to that taxi driver and loving care of the chiropractor, my dad lived long enough to watch me graduate into the profession that gave him a second chance at life, long enough to stand next to me as my best man when I got married, and long enough to meet my first son when he was born. I am blessed beyond measure to have been able to spend an extra 18 quality years with him, the man I respected and loved so much.

Telling you this story explains how I found my passion for chiropractic, the profession that has the power to improve so many lives and help so many people.

Now that you know my story, please answer this question: when my dad was sick and suffering, was he the only one who suffered? Who else was affected? You may say that I, his son suffered, that his whole family did, and that anyone who loved him felt some degree of pain. If that is true, the same goes for you and your family. Therefore our own health should be our first priority. What my sons and my wife want from me is the same thing I wanted most from my father; to be there for them when they need me and to be around for a long time. It's all I wanted from my dad, and it's all your family wants from you.

Here's the point: It's not just about you! If you take your health seriously and if you invest in your wellbeing, you're not doing it just for yourself. You're doing it for your kids and your parents. You're doing it for your spouse and those who love you. Keep that in mind as you continue to read because the way you take care of your health has just as much to do with others as it does with you. And that dear reader, is exactly why I wrote this book.

My hope is that this book provides you with a new perspective in wellness that will become the foundation upon which you build your life. It is also my vision that future generations will look to you as an example and a role model in caring for themselves and their family members.

# Chapter 1
## *What is Stress?*

*"Look deep into nature, and then you will understand everything better."*

-Albert Einstein

# The StressProof Life

One night, when I was seven years old, my parents told me that I had to sleep with the radio on. So, I turned on the radio and turned up the volume. There was no programming on this station and the radio was silent. I quickly fell asleep. Then, after midnight, a loud siren blared through the radio and I frantically flew out of bed. With my parents, we ran out the door, through the hallway, and down the stairs all the way to the basement. Our neighbors from the building were already down there. They were all huddled in groups. Some were talking quietly. Others were praying. The air was heavy with fear.

Suddenly, we heard the deafening roar of a jet engine pass overhead. The noise was so loud that the entire building vibrated. At the same time, we heard the whistle of a bomb that had just been dropped. The people gasped. My mother hugged me tight. The whistle got louder and louder as the bomb got closer and closer. But the sound was so high pitched that we couldn't place it. It could've been right over our heads or it could've been several blocks away and there was no way to tell.

We were petrified and all we could do was helplessly wait, hope, and pray. Then came the loud earthshaking boom of the explosion. The walls of the building trembled and the lights flickered. I squeezed my eyes so tightly shut that I thought they would have to be pried open. Then there was just silence. Not the silence of death, not for the people in our building anyway. We were still alive. We were safe because the bomb had hit a building a block away. The year was 1981 and the place was Tehran, Iran during the Iran-Iraq war.

Can you imagine how we felt hearing that screaming pitch of the bomb as it was falling through the air, not knowing if those were our last moments in this life? *That* was a stressful night for me.

Would you agree that, this type of stress, when experienced night after night could cause a decline in your health?

Stress is relative. Pollution, recession, unemployment, foreclosures, bankruptcies, national debt, Social Security, national healthcare reform, child obesity, internet pornography, new technology, education, retirement, taxes, keeping up with the Joneses...these are all stressors which affect people differently, but ultimately, they all create STRESS!!!

So what is stress? How does it affect us, and how does it affect our health?

In today's world stress is ubiquitous and is quite often blamed for many of the chronic health problems that we face as a society. More than ever before, doctors are citing stress as the source or cause of certain disorders and are prescribing anti-anxiety and anti-depressant medication at record rates.

Those disorders include common conditions such as:

- back pain
- acid reflux
- fibromyalgia
- irritable bowel syndrome
- high blood pressure
- obesity
- and most commonly, headaches

The question to ask would be, can stress really cause health problems such as headaches? And if the answer is yes, we must then ask the more important question of why? Why would stress cause headaches? An even more important question would then be, how can we learn to manage stress in a way that we can prevent such negative health consequences?

## *What is Health?*

In conversations with my patients I have realized that most people's premise on disease and illness is based on incredibly erroneous myths about health and wellness. One such premise is that health is the absence of disease. Consider a man who is moderately overweight with only slightly elevated blood pressure, who cannot climb a set of stairs without running out of breath, does not have the strength to lift a 45lb suitcase, and lacks the flexibility to bend and tie his shoe laces. This man is free of all diseases but given the limitations listed, would you consider him to be *healthy*?

Being healthy is not equal to the absence of disease. Thinking about your health after you've gotten sick, is like putting on your seatbelt after you've crashed your car. Does maintaining dental hygiene require you to only brush and floss your teeth when you have a painful cavity or is it a lifetime process of daily tasks? In the same way, being healthy is a lifestyle and not merely the absence of disease.

Over 90% of diseases are lifestyle diseases and preventable. In fact, Dr. James Chestnut, one of the foremost experts on wellness and human physiology, states that 8 out of 10 people on our continent will die of lifestyle choices. It is disturbing to think that 8 out of every

10 people we know are making choices that are slowing killing them.

Those of us who live in the United States are blessed with the fact that our country is the best in the world in urgent care. We're number one! That means, if you are planning to have a heart attack or a stroke, this is the country to do it in. Isn't that comforting? Basically, as American citizens, we can just relax with absolute peace of mind. Let's not exercise. Let's smoke, let's drink, and let's eat junk food. (Insert sarcasm here!) Let's also volunteer for field duty with the bomb squad and experience the exhilarating thrill of defusing a ticking time bomb. Let's put our trust in the urgent care system. After all it is the best in the world.

If that doesn't sound like the best strategy for healthcare for you and your family, then read on.

Although ninety percent of all diseases are preventable, they aren't being prevented. We know that because each year the numbers keep going up. In fact, between the time I began writing this book and the moment you read it, all of the statistical data on disease prevalence will have changed for the worse. The United States may be number one in urgent care but we are ranked 37th in the world at keeping our citizens healthy, according to the World Health Organization as of 2014.[1] This is in part due to the fact that this country does not have enough *health-care* providers although we have plenty of urgent-care and sick-care providers.

You see, more and more people are now dying from those preventable diseases than ever before. For the first time in history, life expectancy has been decreased [2], which means that our generation is not expected to live as long as the previous generation. It also means that our children will not live as long as we do. Currently there are children and teenagers battling obesity, Type II (adult onset) Diabetes, and degenerative arthritis, all of which used to be old age problems that did not exist in children. I fear that this next generation, our own children will have heart attacks at the age of 30 and it will be considered normal. What in the world is normal about a heart attack, at any age?

If that is not the kind of world you want to live in, and your children to grow up in, then you have to become your own health care providers. You have to take responsibility for your own health. You have to be the one to determine what you do and don't do for your health. I encourage you, be proactive in your own health and lifestyle and in doing so, you can change the future and restore hope for your children and grandchildren. It begins right here, right now.

## *How Does Stress Affect Health?*

So, does stress play a role in our health? The answer is yes, but how? The word stress was coined by Dr. Hans Selye. His work on stress originated from his observation of hospital patients while he was still a student in medical school. In one instance, during Grand Rounds (a teaching tool where medical students are presented with a patient's medical history and problems), one of his professors asked him what he thought was the problem with a particular patient being studied. Hans noticed that although the disease process may have been different, this patient exhibited much of the same signs and symptoms as all the other patients in the hospital. So when asked, "What do you think is wrong with the patient?" Hans answered by saying, this patient "looks sick." At which time, all the interns and residents present began to laugh. Although he was ridiculed for his answer, Dr. Selye knew that he was right. He had observed similarities that were common with all patients no matter what their illness was called.[3] He went on to publish many books and groundbreaking articles on the concept of stress and how the body's response to stress, over time, can result in:

- hormonal imbalance
- high blood pressure
- arteriosclerosis
- arthritis
- kidney disease
- ulcers
- and allergic reactions

His extensive research on the subject of stress proved that most sickness is the result of the body's inability to adapt to stress.

## *How You Handle Stress is a Big Factor in Your Overall Health*

Why is it possible that two different people can be exposed to the same pathogen, the same virus or bacteria, and one will get sick while the other stays symptom-free? Why is it possible that a group of people can eat spoiled food in an unsanitary restaurant and most of them get food poisoning but a select few don't? Why doesn't everyone catch a cold in the winter? If the cause is the same, each body would have the same reaction. If the bacteria are really the cause of the disease, then every person exposed to that bacteria should display the same exact symptoms, in the same exact way, every single time.

What if the truth is that those who display symptoms, those who get sick, were actually already sick? Don't just gloss over that question, but really think about it. What if we are wrong about what we define as being sick?

An experiment was once performed where two groups of people were injected with the flu virus.[4] I'm not sure how they encouraged these people to volunteer for this study, but the results were astonishing.

The first group of subjects was comprised of type A, highly driven, career-focused people. They were the type of people who could be termed workaholics. They worked very long hours, spent very little time in leisure, and rarely went on vacations. For lack of a better term, their lives were out of balance. The second group consisted of individuals who balanced their time between work and play. These people were in committed relationships and took time to spend with family and friends. They also made time for regular social events and were involved in organizations outside of their profession.

When the first group was injected with the flu virus, the subjects were bed-ridden for several days. They suffered from a spectrum of symptoms such as sinus congestion, runny nose, cough, headache, and joint aches. On the other hand when the second group was injected with the same flu virus, in the same exact way, the individuals hardly showed any symptoms. Why is that?

I hope you're ready for the answer: the first group was already sick. This is profound because it was their lifestyle that over time had reduced their ability to handle stress. The truth is that both groups contracted the flu but the second group had unwittingly StressProofed their lives which rendered them able to deal with it much better than the first group.

Have you ever wondered, where the flu virus goes in the summer? Is the flu virus like a goose that likes to fly north for the summer and south for the winter? Is it like a bear that likes to hibernate, except it hibernates in the summer instead of the winter? Is it like an owl that sleeps during the day and wakes up when it's dark, except the flu virus sleeps when it's warm and only wakes up when it's cold? The fact is that the flu virus does not migrate, does not hibernate, and isn't too concerned about the weather outside. It is always present, day and night, summer and winter. Haven't you ever heard of someone catching a cold or the flu in the summer?

Think about Dr. Hans Selye's research on stress. His focus was not on the stress but the body's response to stress. One of the stresses that we must deal with in the winter is cold weather. The human body must maintain its core temperature at 98.6 degrees and if the outside temperature is less than that, the body is placed under stress. Therefore the body must work to bring the core temperature up to its ideal level. The colder it gets, the harder the body must work. Therefore, cold weather is a stressor; it is a source of stress.

Is it not true that people handle stress differently? In some individuals stress will cause a weakened immune system which leads to contraction of colds and flu. In some individuals stress will cause a heart attack or a stroke. In others it will cause heartburn, acid reflux, or indigestion. Still in some individuals stress will cause tension headaches or migraine headaches.

It is time for a major paradigm shift in how we view health. We have to accept that the person who "catches" a cold was already sick. The one who "contracts" the flu was already sick. The one who has a heart attack was already sick. You and I may be sick already.

A highly respected colleague once used an analogy to illustrate this concept. He said that vultures do not kill animals. They only show up when the animal is already dead. In the same way, many classes of bugs, bacteria, and viruses can't really hurt people in small amounts but they do like to multiply and infiltrate when the body is weak.

An example of this would be streptococcal bacteria. Strep can be found in practically every human being but not every human being currently has a sore throat or strep throat. It only becomes a disease when there is an overgrowth of the strep bacteria, and this overgrowth can only occur if the body is weak and allows it to happen.

Another similar example would be Candida Albicans which cause yeast infections. These microorganisms are always present but an overgrowth will cause sickness.

A third example would be fungal infections. You get the point.

I am not stating that the old concept of the germ theory is incorrect. I am just pointing out that it is incomplete, meaning it fails to explain why the same germ (bacteria/pathogen) does not cause the same exact symptoms in every human body in the same exact way and according to the same exact timeline.

For the germ theory to be considered a law, the germ should cause the same illness, in the same way, every single time. The majority of the common pathogens and germs are very opportunistic in nature and only take advantage of the weak. There are only a minority of pathogens that are so deadly that they do behave in a predictable way. Even so, consider 2014's Ebola outbreak. Ebola is one of the deadliest viruses known. Even the name of the virus is terrifying. Yet, more than half of those who contracted the virus made a full recovery.[5] According to the germ theory none should have survived. Why do you think everyone didn't die?

We must stop believing that there is always one cause and one cure for each disease. If the disease manifests differently in different people there must be a reason for it and therefore we must discard the monocausal approach to the treatment of disease. There are multiple causes to every disease and one of those that must be considered in every case is the individual's ability or inability to adapt to stress. So, stress is bad, right?

## Life Without Stress

One of my favorite stories about stress is about Dr. Norman Vincent Peale. He was the author of the best-selling book *The Power of Positive Thinking*. In one instance, he was in his office with a client and this client was going on and on about how much stress he was under and how the stress in his life was to blame for everything that went wrong in his world. He stated that he wished he didn't have any stress. After listening intently to this man, Dr. Peale asked, "Would you like to meet some people who don't have any stress?" To this question the gentleman gave a resounding and enthusiastic "*Yes!*" He stated that he would absolutely love to meet them and find out what they do for a living and how they deal with their family and finances. Dr. Peale said, "We can go meet some of them right now, follow me." The gentleman followed Dr. Peale as he walked out of the door of his office, down the corridor, out the front doors of the church, across the parking lot, and onto the cemetery. Dr. Peale pointed to the headstones and graves and said "These are the people who don't have any stress."

Researchers in a laboratory wanted to know what happens to living organisms when devoid of all stress. They used single-cell organisms called amoeba for this research. They placed the amoeba in an environment that was perfect for them. The temperature was perfect and they were provided with just the right amount of nutrients – not too much and not too little. What the researchers noticed was astonishing. The cells all failed to thrive and every one of them died prematurely.[6]

So, these researchers would agree with Dr. Peale. Being stress-free is equivalent to death. Let's get this straight. Stress can cause heart disease, stroke, cancer, headaches, heartburn, ulcers, and suppress our immune system, yet without stress we die. So, is stress good or bad?

## Stress, Good or Bad?

Let's define the word stress. Dr. Hans Selye defined stress as "the non-specific response of the body to any demand placed on it." Dr. Patrick Gentempo and Dr. Christopher Kent, cofounders of the Chiropractic Leadership Alliance, define stress as "a force that causes change in your life." Notice that the definition of stress doesn't state that it is a negative force that causes change in life. The definition also doesn't state that the changes caused by the force are always negative.

The fact is that your health is dependent on how well you handle stress. Actually, your success in life and in any endeavor is also entirely dependent on how well and how much stress you can handle. Therefore, the goal should never be to reduce or eliminate stress. Especially since elimination of stress is equivalent to dying. Our goal should be to reduce the probability of a **negative response** to stress.

You see, just as people handle germs differently, people also handle stress differently. Two people can be under equal stress. One person will have a heart attack as a result of that stress and the other won't have any ill effect. Which would you rather be? One person may have a stroke and the other will not. Which would you rather be? One may develop high blood pressure, ulcers, intestinal irritability, hormonal irregularity, headaches, and depression while the other may not develop any of these things. Which person would you like to be?

Asking if stress if good or bad is like asking if gravity is good or bad. Or asking if money is good or bad. What about fire? Starting a new business, obtaining higher education, expanding your family with children, chasing your dreams, all have varying degrees of stress. Are they good or bad? Stress is neither good nor bad, just as gravity, money, and fire are neither good nor bad.

Arnold Schwarzenegger attributes his life's success to the strength he developed by lifting weights. My patient Bob attributes his herniated disc to the same physical act of lifting weights in a gym. Does that mean lifting weights is good, or is it bad?

According to a Forbes magazine Special Report entitled "America's 50 Top Givers", in 2013, William Baron Hilton donated 92 million dollars to support his passion for ending homelessness in Los Angeles. On the other hand Osama

Bin Laden spent millions of dollars in preparation for the September 11 attack on the United States. Does that mean money is a good thing, or is it bad?

The important concept to understand is that stress is only the force and the body is responsible for responding to that force. The body can respond in a positive way by becoming stronger and healthier, or it can respond in a negative way by becoming weaker and eventually ill. This is known as the body's adaptation potential.

Each person has a different level of adaptability to stress. Imagine a paper cup placed upside down on a table. How much weight do you think it can handle? Can I place a small paperback book on it and expect it to hold? How about a large hardcover encyclopedia? How about two, three, or four large heavy books? Eventually the cup will succumb to the weight of the books and it will collapse. What if I use a metal cup instead of the paper cup? Will it collapse under the same amount of weight (stress) or will it be able to hold much more weight before bending? Which cup would you rather be? A cup is inanimate but the human body has the ability to adapt. The body's adaptation potential is what determines how much stress someone can handle before they succumb to illness.

Earlier I mentioned that our goal should not be to reduce stress but to reduce the probability of a negative response to stress. Stated differently, our goal should be to increase the body's adaptation potential. That is how we can StressProof ourselves against the possibility of a negative response to stress.

As we increase the body's adaptation potential, not only do we reduce the probability of a negative response to stress, but we also increase the probability of a positive response to stress. What are some examples of a positive response to stress?

One example is increased self-esteem and self-confidence. As our ability to handle stress increases, a natural response is strength of character and knowing that you can handle what challenges may come your way.

It's been said that most multi-millionaires have been bankrupt at least once prior to becoming wealthy. As they overcome past challenges, the stress of a financial hardship may actually create emotions of motivation, enthusiasm, and optimism instead of fear, dismay, and depression. Which set of emotions would be more conducive to success? The person with the former set of emotions has a higher adaptation potential to financial stress.

I know business owners who, under financial stress, have packed up their bags, shut down their doors, and walked away from their dreams. I also know business owners who during tough times have stood their ground, found ways to innovate, and as a result, built businesses that can weather most financial storms. Who do you think had better adaptability to stress?

In the same way a child who has contracted and overcome Chickenpox, now has immunity against this virus and will no longer become ill when exposed to it. Those who do not get chickenpox at childhood are at risk of a more serious illness as an adult when exposed to the same virus.

## *The Three Dimensions of Stress*

A common mistake people make when thinking about stress is that most people think of it only in emotional or psychological terms. However, stress can present itself in three different dimensions. The three dimensions of stress are physical, chemical, and psychological.

## Physical Stress

Here are some examples of stress in the physical dimension that can have a negative impact on your health:

- Sitting with poor posture
- Spending long hours in front of a computer
- Poor ergonomics at work
- Improper lifting
- Sleeping on an old sagging mattress
- Contact sports
- Over-training for athletes
- Car accidents
- Slip-and-falls
- Other traumatic injuries
- Process of birth
- Learning to walk

As I mentioned earlier, the body's response to stress is much more important than the stress itself. You see, exercise is a stress and if done properly it will lead to a positive response in the body. Resistance training with weights or bands can lead to stronger muscles and joints. Cardiovascular exercise from running, swimming, or skiing can result in improved heart and lung function and lead to better health. One can put stress on their muscles through weight lifting and their muscles will grow but another person can put the same stress on their muscles and get injured. The results are entirely dependent on the person's adaptability to the specific stress. If a novice weight-lifter attempts to bench press 300 pounds on his first day at the gym, he or she will be seriously injured. An experienced and properly trained power-lifter will have no difficulties doing the same exercise. Our focus should always be on the body's response to stress and not the stress itself.

Chemical Stress

How do chemicals affect our stress response? What we breathe in, what we ingest, and what we absorb through our skin are all stressors in the body, but they can either produce a negative result or a positive result. Sources of stress in the chemical dimension include:

- Air pollution
- Water pollution
- Cigarette smoke
- Second hand smoke
- Work-related hazardous materials
- Asbestos
- Antiperspirants
- Some deodorants
- Perfumes/colognes
- Drugs
- Food preservatives
- Pesticides
- Herbicides
- Cleaning agents
- Dryer sheets
- And the list goes on

Looking at this list it might seem commonsense that these items are harmful, but consider the following. Breathing oxygen typically results in a positive response by the body, but if you hyperventilate, you could pass out. Drinking pure, clean water is good for you but drink an excessive amount of water and the resulting electrolyte imbalance can be detrimental to your health and even fatal. The same applies to certain vitamins and foods. We will discuss vitamins later. The point again is that the body's response to stress is much more important than the source of stress.

Consider cigarette smoking. This is a stress that is detrimental to your health in any amount. The lungs are damaged by only one puff of smoke and each subsequent puff of smoke that is inhaled will add to that damage. However, one person may smoke a pack per day for decades and never experience lung disease while another person may smoke a pack a day for just 10 years and develop terminal lung cancer.

Joan Schiller, MD (Professor and Chief of Hematology/Oncology at Southwestern Medical Center) writes: "So why don't all smokers get lung cancer? Several reasons. First, one needs to accumulate a lot of these mutations before the cell becomes cancerous. Secondly, for reasons we do not completely understand, some people seem to be more susceptible to getting mutations from these cancer-causing substances than others. Finally, our bodies are remarkably good at repairing the mutations when they do happen, so in many cases they never cause the cell to become cancerous."[7]

As you can see there is never just one cause for each disease. Many different factors play a role in the disease process. The person who developed cancer after smoking one pack a day for several years may also have had some vitamin deficiencies and maybe he was also obese. Perhaps in addition to smoking he had a bad drinking habit, was in the middle of a divorce and fighting for custody of his children. These scenarios create an extreme picture but any one of these situations would most definitely reduce the person's ability to adapt to stress. Would he have gotten lung cancer if he was otherwise in great mental and physical health? We will never know. However, we can state with great certainty, that the chances of getting cancer would be less.

## Psychological Stress

That brings us to the psychological dimension of stress. Anything that can create an emotional change is considered psychological stress. The change can be positive or negative. For example an argument with your spouse would be a stress that may cause a negative emotion. In the same relationship, intimately connecting with your spouse will result in a host of positive emotions.

Working in a job that you dislike will result in negative emotions. Working toward a goal that excites you will result in positive emotions. The stressor in this example is work, but the psychological response can vary drastically.

Dealing with financial hardship during an economic recession and worries about job security will result in a negative response to stress. Starting a new business that is phenomenally successful, provides abundantly for your family, and produces a venue for you to express your gifts and talents will most definitely produce a positive emotional state.

## *Wellness Requires You to Improve All Three Dimensions Simultaneously*

To truly achieve wellness, you should improve yourself in all three dimensions of stress simultaneously. This doesn't need to be a difficult nor drastic endeavor. If you begin to exercise properly but neglect your life in the chemical and psychological dimensions, you may not achieve true wellness. If you begin to eat a balanced and nutritious diet, and at the same time, not exercise, and not improve your thought-life (the way you think), you won't attain true wellness. Certainly, if you begin to eliminate negative emotions from your psychological dimension and expect to achieve wellness without improving your dietary habits and physical rituals you will again be disappointed. But it isn't difficult to improve all three at the same time. Because, if you make only small changes in each dimension and do them simultaneously, you will experience noticeable improvement in your overall level of wellness.

I know many people who exercise on a regular basis and some of them even eat an extremely well balanced and nutritious diet, yet still haven't reached their goals in health and fitness. That is because they haven't been addressing all three dimensions of stress and health simultaneously.

Here is a good example of someone who made small changes and saw noticeable results.

Robert was overweight, complained of chronic back pain, and battled depression. In the physical dimension he changed the pillow and mattress that he slept on at night and began to exercise by going up and down the stairs in his house for 10 minutes every morning. In the chemical dimension he chose to stop taking pain killers and instead addressed his back problems through chiropractic care. He also increased the amount of water he drank and reduced the amount of diet soda he was drinking. In the psychological dimension, he decided that he would pray for 10 minutes every day in a quiet place. He also began a collection of jokes and kept a journal in which he wrote down the funniest jokes he would hear. His friends and coworkers would constantly bring him new jokes and he would write them down. This caused him to laugh out loud several times each day. His back pain disappeared, he lost weight, and he no longer battled depression. He now plans to write two books, one about his transformation, and the other is a collection of his favorite jokes. Small changes in all three dimensions of life, if done simultaneously, will have a significant impact in your overall level of wellness.

## *So What Is Wellness?*

There are "Wellness Centers" popping up all over the country. It's now a buzz word and marketers are having a field day with it. You can see wellness pharmacies and wellness hospitals everywhere. Massage therapists, acupuncturists, chiropractors, and nutritionists are all calling themselves wellness practitioners. How do they all define wellness? More importantly how do you measure your level of wellness? When do you know you have achieved wellness?

These are very important questions and they must be answered in order for us to know how to change for the better. If we don't know what wellness is, how do we know if we're headed in the right direction?

According to the Creating Wellness Alliance, wellness is the degree in which health and vitality are experienced in every dimension of life. You see, by definition, wellness is not a destination. It's a direction. It's like traveling east or traveling west. There is no limit to the amount of wellness you can achieve.

Wellness and illness exist on a continuum. Visualize yourself standing with your arms spread as far apart as possible, with your right index finger pointing to the right and your left index finger pointing to the left. Let this represent the wellness continuum. Assume the right index finger is pointing toward wellness and the left index finger is pointing toward illness. Your body represents where you currently stand on that continuum. The important thing to remember is that the body is never static. It is constantly moving in one of two directions. It is either moving toward wellness or away from wellness and toward illness. Every thought, action, and decision you make moves you in one of these two directions. Your daily choices are constantly pushing you back and forth on the vast spectrum of wellness and illness. You cannot move toward wellness and illness simultaneously, just as you cannot be traveling east and west simultaneously.

Dr. Patrick Gentempo, the founder of the Creating Wellness Alliance, asks this question of his audience when speaking about wellness. "Can you think of just one thing that you could be doing, that you're currently not doing, that would move you in the direction of wellness?" He has never gotten a "no" as the answer to that question. We can always think of at least one thing that we could do differently to move further in the direction of wellness. The next question Dr. Gentempo asks is, "Why aren't you doing it?" That question usually seems a bit harder to answer. I know that my typical answer would be that I don't have the time to do it. If that is your answer too, then you and I should sit down and re-evaluate our priorities. If you want to be healthier, this is the first requirement. If our time is limited and every minute of our time is already accounted for, then we must choose to take time away from something and dedicate it to improving our level of wellness.

Dr. Gentempo would say that you don't need a "To-Do list," you need a "To-Don't list." Make a list of things you don't need to keep doing and free up some time. Do you need to keep reading every email in your spam box? Do you need to aimlessly surf the internet after you're done reading your email? Do you need to keep playing solitaire on your smart phone? Do you need to spend the next half hour on the phone with your best friend complaining about how you never have time to do anything?

Like I said, to move in the direction of wellness, it's time to reevaluate our priorities. What do you value the most in life? Is it your family? Is it your health? Is it your career? Is it your church? Do you value education? Do you value entertainment? One way to find out exactly what your core values are is to look at your checkbook. How do you spend your money? After your mortgage and bills, what do you write the biggest checks to? If you spend your discretionary income on movies and theater, your core value could be entertainment. If you spend it on books and seminars, your core values include education. Take a moment and determine what your true core values are.

You may determine that what you truly value isn't something you actually want to value. For example, if you find out that most of your discretionary income is spent in restaurants, it would mean that you place substantial value on either dining out or the social interaction of dining out. The truth is that we give our money to the things we value most. What are your core values?

As a doctor, I regularly meet people who say that one of their core values is health and wellness. Yet when we discuss this further, we discover that very little of their resources, time and money are being spent on being healthy and well. If you spend your valuable time reading this book, then health is of value to you. All you have to do now is link it to your bigger core values. If family is your biggest core value, then consider that you can be a better parent, a better spouse, a better sibling, and a better friend if you are healthier. If your career and profession are also top core values, then link them to health and wellness by accepting the fact that you can be a better employee, a better boss, a better leader, a better producer, and a better provider for your family if you are healthier.

Can you enjoy life more if you are healthier? Can you enjoy your vacations more if you are healthier? Can you enjoy your hobbies and pursue your passions more if you are healthier? If yes, then make health and wellness a priority.

Now that we agree that health and wellness should be a core value and of high priority, we must then answer the question, how do we ensure that we allocate the proper amount of time, money and energy to our core priorities? Also, since we are speaking about stress, how do we manage all this without decreasing our ability to handle the stress?

Contemplating that question reminds me of a story that I read in a forwarded email. You may have seen and read this story before and you may have heard it many times but it is worth repeating as its message directly impacts how we view our life with regard to stress.

The story is about a college professor teaching an important lesson to his philosophy students on the first day of class. The professor placed an empty glass jar on the podium and told his students "Consider that this jar is completely empty." He pulled out a basket of golf balls from beneath the podium and proceeded to fill the jar until he could not fit another golf ball into the jar. He asked his students if the jar was now full. The students said yes. The professor then pulled out a cup that was filled with pebbles and began pouring the pebbles into the jar. The pebbles fell into and filled the space between the golf balls. The professor then asked again, "How about now, is the jar full?" The students again said yes. So, the professor picked up a cup of sand and proceeded to pour the sand into the jar. The sand filled in the space in between the pebbles and golf balls and filled the jar to the rim. At this point, the students all agreed that now the jar was definitely full. At which time the professor brought out two cups of tea and poured them into the jar. The tea seeped into the jar and took up space between the grains of sand, the pebbles and the golf balls and the students laughed.

When the laughter stopped, the professor explained to the students that the glass jar represented their life. He said that we all have a finite amount of space in our jars. The golf balls represent our main priorities. They represent God, our families, our children, our health, etc. The pebbles are the other significant concerns of our life. They represent our jobs, our education, our houses, our cars, etc. The sand represents the insignificant things in life like watching TV, reading the comics, doing a jigsaw puzzle, etc. If we first fill our jar with sand we won't have room to put the golf balls in. If we allow our lives to be filled with the insignificant things, there won't be any room for what's really important.

Then a student asked the professor what the tea was representative of. To this, the professor answered, "no matter how busy you are, you always have time for a cup of tea with a friend."

So, what are you starting with? Do you schedule prioritized time to spend with your family? Or, do you fill your time with pebbles and if there's something left over, then you spend it with family? Do you schedule your exercise time in advance, or do you say "I'll get to it when I get to it?" What if you scheduled your family time and workouts the same way you schedule your business meetings and your doctor's appointments? Have you ever made an appointment with yourself? It sounds a bit silly at first but if you need 30 minutes per day to be alone in quiet so that you can manage your thoughts, why not schedule it in advance and block out the time like an actual appointment? If health is one of your golf balls, and it should be, then you have to intentionally place it in the jar before the pebbles and the sand.

If you are still reading, then I assume that you have decided to make wellness one of your golf balls, and you have made a commitment to StressProof your life. I congratulate you.

You should be thinking, "Okay, I now know the definition of stress, its three dimensions, and that wellness is achieved by improving the three dimensions simultaneously. Now please tell me what I need to do to StressProof my life."

Not just yet! In the same way that we discussed the new paradigm of stress, we need to discuss two other concepts. I call them 'The Genius of Genetics' and 'The Beauty of the Brain'. Once you have gained a basic understanding of these concepts you will be ready to receive exact instructions on how to fully StressProof your life.

So, without further delay, please join me in taking an exciting new look at the genius of your genetics. It is the next stop on our voyage of discovery, exploring the secrets to creating a StressProof life.

Sources:

1. ABC source "World Health Organization Assesses the World's Health Systems."*WHO*. N.p., n.d. Web. 04 June 2015.

2. Geier, Kathleen. "Shocker Stat of the Day: Life Expectancy Decreases by 4 Years among Poor White People in the U.S." *The Washington Monthly*. N.p., 22 Sept. 2012. Web. 01 July 2014.

3. Selye, Hans. *The Stress of Life (Paperback Edition)*. N.p.: n.p., 1978. Print.

4. Ortberg, John. "Everybody's Normal 'Til You Get to Know Them." Zondervan, 2003

5. Diamond, Dan. "The Ebola Number You Haven't Heard: 80% Of U.S. Ebola Patients Have Survived." *Forbes*. Forbes Magazine, 21 Oct. 2014. Web

6. Ortberg, John. "Everybody's Normal 'Til You Get to Know Them." Zondervan, 2003

7. Schiller, Joan, M.D. "Cancer Q&A | Why Do Some Smokers Never Get Lung Cancer, and Others Who Don't Smoke End up Getting It?" UT Southwestern Medical Center. N.p., 2011. Web

# Chapter 2
# *The Genius of Genetics, the Blueprint of Life*

*"It is a single cell's "awareness" of the environment, not its genes, that sets into motion the mechanism of life."*

- Bruce H. Lipton, Ph.D.

My patient Herbert was only 68 years old when he died. He died of pancreatic cancer. I absolutely loved being Herbert's chiropractor for the last 10 years of his life. He was a heavy-set man, somewhat overweight with graying brown hair, and he stood about six feet tall. He was a man of few words but every word was always chosen with purpose. He was an attorney but didn't practice law in the traditional sense. He worked for a large corporation and handled the legal aspects of the business. He was exceptionally intelligent and knowledgeable which made him a great conversationalist. He was also extremely kind and always took the time to ask about my family. He would frequently make helpful suggestions for my next vacation or how to entertain my family better.

Approximately six years before he died, he was diagnosed with terminal pancreatic cancer. His doctor told him that he had less than a year to live and that he should get his affairs in order.

Herbert retired from his job and decided to take a trip to Southeast Asia. He always wanted to go there but had never made time to do so. He spent 6 weeks traveling and had a great time. The cancer treatment seemed to be working because Herbert felt fine and although the cancer had spread to his spine, the tumors were growing very slowly. He was in good spirits and regularly talked about how he was "on borrowed time and enjoying it."

A few months before he passed, his oncologist started him on another round of chemotherapy. Two months later, after the chemotherapy was done, the doctor ordered a new CT scan of his chest, abdomen, and spine. The scan showed that the cancer was severely advanced and that he had multiple new tumors in the lungs, liver, pancreas, and spine. They told Herbert that he probably only had a few days left to live.

I saw Herbert the day after he heard this news. For the first time he actually looked sick. Don't get me wrong. He had been losing a lot of weight and he certainly didn't have the physical stature that he had 10 years ago but for the first time since his cancer diagnosis 6 years prior, he actually looked the part of a cancer patient. It was shocking to see how rapidly he deteriorated the minute they told him that he was near the end. He told me he was going to stop all treatments except for his chiropractic care. He passed away a week later. I wonder if he would have lived longer if the doctors hadn't told him how sick he really was on the inside. I really miss Herbert.

The reason I share this story is because most experts have told us that cancer has a strong genetic component and that's the central focus of this chapter.

As long as we are alive, our bodies will continue to repair, regenerate, and regulate themselves. It's absolutely miraculous when you think about it. Our bodies are made up of cells. Cells are the basic unit of life. There are various different types of cells that comprise the human body and each type of cell has a different function. Some cells self-replicate and others are produced by different cells. Cell biology (the study of life) makes a valiant attempt to explain how these cells function.

However, the fields of biology, chemistry and physics can only provide a limited explanation of life. Through observation, they can describe the processes of life but they fail to explain how such processes are controlled and organized. This means there are irreducible complexities that have remained unexplainable through conventional science. As a result, many scientists have chosen to refer to the aggregate of these complexities as inborn wisdom or innate intelligence.

This is evident in the fact that technology hasn't figured out how to create life from inanimate resources. What I mean is that we may be able to build a mechanical model of a cell and build so much detail into it that it can actually work like a regular human cell. Perhaps it will have an outer barrier like the cell membrane that allows for nutrients to come in and waste product to be excreted. Perhaps it has a power plant like the cell mitochondria which generates energy to power the cell. It can even have a program blueprint like DNA that instructs the cell how to function in different environments. The one thing we cannot do is get that cell to become self-healing and self-replicating. Current scientific technology cannot use nonliving material to build a cell that is alive. Our cells use food to rebuild, repair and regenerate parts of themselves. The laws of physics and chemistry cannot explain this phenomenon. Yet no one can dispute the fact that living cells possess an intrinsic healing power.

Think about the origin of a human life. We know that approximately 300 million sperm are released into the birth canal and one of those sperm cells will fertilize the egg. Studying the process we can observe exactly what happens in each phase of fertilization but we don't know exactly how the 23 chromosomes from the sperm unite with the 23 chromosomes from the egg to create a zygote which then develops into a ball of stem cells.

Furthermore, we know that those stem cells will differentiate into different body parts but we don't know exactly what makes one of those stem cells develop into a brain cell and another into a bone, skin or eye cell.

While all that is happening inside the womb, the pregnant mother begins to experience morning sickness. She is genetically preprogrammed to respond this way. Have you ever wondered why? And why it is that some women have worse symptoms than others? Is it really a sickness, or is it actually an expression of health? Throughout history, whenever morning sickness was chemically interfered with, the outcome was not favorable.

During the 1950's and possibly earlier, a drug called Thalidomide was prescribed to pregnant women for morning sickness. Birth defects resulted when medication was used to suppress the nausea of morning sickness. This bears the question, did the drug cause the birth defects or did suppressing morning sickness result in the malformation of body parts in the babies? I don't know the answer but if I had to guess, I would say, probably both!

I believe, it is dangerous to artificially suppress morning sickness and it is equally as dangerous to put synthetic pharmaceuticals into the body during any stage of pregnancy. Both approaches can and will interfere with the genetic development of the baby.[1,2]

The American College of Obstetrics & Gynecology published in 2000 the following statement:

"Morning sickness has been reported to have a positive effect on pregnancy outcome and is associated with a decreased risk of miscarriage, preterm birth, low birth weight, and perinatal death."[3]

This article further stated that lower nutrient intake, as caused by the nausea and vomiting of morning sickness, actually causes the placenta to develop normally. A study of malnourished women in the Dutch Famine Study revealed that the children of women who were malnourished during all three trimesters were of lower than normal birth weight, but those women who experienced malnourishment only during their first trimester of pregnancy gave birth to babies of healthy weight. In conclusion, being malnourished during the first trimester of pregnancy, whether it is caused by morning sickness or a famine, is a good thing as evidenced by the birth of healthy babies. Perhaps their mothers are genetically programmed to experience morning sickness in order to protect their babies.

So if morning sickness actually helps to produce healthy babies, is it really sickness? Could this be another example of the intrinsic wisdom of life that knows exactly what to do? Perhaps we should begin calling it morning wellness instead of morning sickness.

Then there's the matter of weird cravings during pregnancy. Suddenly my wife was saying that her favorite foods now make her nauseated but foods like fish that she previously disliked, she was now craving. Could it be that the innate wisdom of her body and her genetic programming was telling her that in this stage of development, her favorite food was actually bad for the baby but fish was needed? This is yet another reason why it is dangerous to chemically interfere with morning sickness using drugs.

It is miraculous how the body knows exactly what to do when devoid of interference.

The innate intelligence does not stop working after the baby is born. Consider the young child. What if he begins to feel nausea? Would you think he is sick or would you say he is healthy? The nausea could be because he put something in his mouth that should not have been ingested. His body has decided that the substance needs to come out. It will create the sensation of nausea and begin to vomit until every bit of the harmful substance has been expelled. Then the nausea will disappear and the child will feel fine. He is genetically programmed to respond this way.

Doesn't the same thing happen when someone drinks too much alcohol? The wisdom of the body decides that vomiting the alcohol out of the stomach is much healthier than allowing the alcohol to enter the blood stream and cause severe alcohol poisoning. How does the stomach know that more alcohol would be so harmful? How does it know that the liquid in the stomach is alcohol and not water or juice? Therefore in this case vomiting is not a sign of sickness, but an expression of health.

Why would a perfectly healthy child suddenly get diarrhea? Similar to vomiting, the body is choosing to expel something that is harmful. Perhaps it was something that the child put in his mouth and vomiting wasn't able to get rid of it. Now it has passed through the stomach and is in the intestinal tract. Certainly, the child should be monitored closely and the child's pediatrician should be notified, but under most circumstances, the condition should be allowed to run its course. When the pathogen is out of the body, the child will naturally stop having diarrhea. Isn't the wisdom of the body miraculous? Once again, in this case, the diarrhea is not a sign of sickness but an expression of health.

What does the innate wisdom of the body choose to do if the pathogen enters the body not through the mouth but through the nose and into the respiratory tract? You guessed it. The child will in this case either cough or sneeze. What if that is not enough to get rid of the pathogen? Then the child will continue to cough until his body decides that all of the "bad guys" are out of his body. If repeated coughing fails to get everything out, then his body will produce mucous to trap the "foreigners" and then he will cough up the mucous and thus get rid of the unwanted substances in the respiratory tract. What would happen if unwanted bacteria were to enter the lungs and the child didn't cough? Who is the healthier child, the one who coughs or the one who doesn't?

Why would a healthy child get a fever? The body is genetically programmed to do whatever it takes to maintain its temperature at 98.6 degrees Fahrenheit. If it's 30 degrees outside, the body works hard to bring the body temperature up to 98.6 and when it's 100 degrees outside, the body works in the opposite direction to bring the body temperature down to 98.6. Why then would it suddenly raise the temperature higher? Body temperature isn't something that randomly occurs but is closely monitored and carefully regulated by the innate intelligence. So, when a child spikes a fever, it means his body suddenly decided that it must work even harder and expend even more energy to generate more heat. Why? You're probably thinking "Because the fever is a sign of some type of infection." That is correct, but does this mean that the child is sick or is he healthy?

Earlier we said that healthy kids vomit, and healthy kids get diarrhea, and healthy kids cough. The wisdom of the body, its innate intelligence and genetic programming are at work to cleanse and protect the body. Does the same apply to fevers?

Allow me to answer that with an illustration. If you were thirsty and stranded in the wilderness would you drink water from a pond or a lake? Or, would you boil the water first before you drank it? Those who are avid campers and have had wilderness training will typically say that you shouldn't drink the water without first boiling it. The act of boiling the water will kill all bacteria and render the water safe to drink. In the human body, the fever is doing the same thing as boiling the water. It knows in its infinite wisdom that the harmful virus or overgrowth of bacteria cannot survive in higher temperatures. Therefore the fever will cycle up and down until every last one of the "bugs" are dead. Once it is certain that the coast is clear, the body will then normalize its temperature back to, you guessed it, 98.6 degrees.

All fevers must be monitored by the child's physician or chiropractor, but think twice before throwing a fever reducer in at the first sign of an elevated reading on the thermometer.

It's obvious that the body has a pre-written program that it runs on. Like a computer, the body is pre-programmed to respond in a certain way to each stimulus. This program is the human DNA. According to Dr. Bruce Lipton, the author of *The Biology of Belief,* your DNA is the blueprint that your cells use to become you. Your DNA determines the color of your eyes, the color of your skin, the color of your hair, and your gender.

DNA is unique to each individual, which is why it can be used during a criminal investigation to determine whether a suspect is guilty based on DNA found at the scene of the crime. Unless you have an identical twin, no one in the world has the same DNA as you. Genes are segments of your DNA that contain information for a specific bodily function or characteristic. So in theory, if we analyze your genetics we should be able to predict exactly what your strengths and weaknesses are going to be, what diseases you will battle in life, and how long you are going to live. But in actuality this statement couldn't be further from the truth.

That exact theory was the mission of the Human Genome Project, to completely map out the human DNA in order to not only predict diseases in advance but to devise interventions that would prevent such diseases. One of the realizations of this project as reported in the New York Times was that humans are all 99.9% identical.[4] I find this fascinating. If you and I are 99.9% identical, why do we look, feel, and act so differently and why don't we respond to stress the same exact way? This includes people of the opposite sex. It states that even men and woman are 99.9% genetically identical. Then where do our differences come from?

All of our body parts develop from stem cells. The human embryo is a ball of stem cells. Every one of those cells contains the exact same DNA. Then why do they differentiate into so many different body parts? If my hair cells have the same DNA as my skin cells, then why do they look and behave so differently? All of our body parts were the same at one point, but something in their environment activated a gene inside that cell that made the cell start to differentiate. This is the exact reason stem cell research is so fascinating and at the same time so controversial. Scientists have discovered that if you remove stem cells from a fetus and place them next to a living organ of another human being, those cells differentiate into that exact organ. So, if you place stem cells next to a live pancreas, they become pancreatic cells and if you put them next to a liver they become hepatic (liver) cells. So then it isn't the genetics of the cell that determines what that cell becomes. It is the environment of the cell that determines which genes get expressed in that specific cell. How important then is it for us to protect our cellular environment?

Another discovery of the Human Genome Project was that there are actually 20,000 genes in the human DNA but approximately 100,000 different genetic characteristics. When the Project was completed in 2003, the 20,000 genes could not begin to explain the 100,000 different expressions of genes. The natural conclusion, according to Dr. Bruce Lipton, is that each gene can express itself in different ways.

In his book, Dr. Lipton talks about research performed with genetically identical Agouti mice. One group of pregnant mice was given folic acid, vitamin B12, betaine, and choline while the other group of genetically identical pregnant mice was fed a diet without these supplements. The mice who were given the supplements produced offspring that were brown in color, physically lean, and had a significantly reduced incidence of obesity, diabetes, and cancer as compared to their genetically identical counterparts who were obese, diabetic, and had a yellow coat. How could genetically identical mice be so extremely different? The supplements must have changed their cellular environment, causing their genes to be expressed differently.

Chances are that, like me, you grew up believing that your genes are the determining factor of your health. In school, we were told that we all have DNA which creates a specific code for our body and health. We believed that if our parents encountered heart disease, or cancer, or diabetes, that it is in our genetic make-up and that we are predestined to also encounter those illnesses. We were told that there is not much we can do about it. How does that make you feel?

The human body has between 50 and 75 trillion cells. Each cell contains the same DNA. So, if someone is born with the gene for cancer then why isn't that person born with the cancer already manifested? Why is it that it unpredictably and suddenly appears later in life? And, why is it that some people with cancer in their genes don't ever get cancer?

The answer is that our genetic code for certain characteristics and tendencies is similar to having a blueprint from which a house could be built. The blueprint contains all the elements that make up the structure, but the plans have to be read by an architect to actually build the house. The architect must interpret the plans in order for the final product to be created. We are all genetically preprogrammed to cough, sneeze, vomit, and spike fevers but we don't walk around all day and every day doing those things. Only if something in our environment triggers the preprogrammed genetic response will the architect of the body read and activate those programs.

So you may ask, why then do so many people with a family gene for cancer often develop cancer? To explore this concept let's look at how cancer research is performed in laboratories. Mice are an excellent subject for studying genetic and hereditary causes of cancer because, through inbreeding or genetically altering the mice, the researchers can easily replicate the type of cancer they are investigating. According to the National Cancer Institute, when these mice are exposed to a known "carcinogen or a cancer-causing agent," they characteristically develop malignant tumors. The predictability of their response makes these mice ideal for studying cancer. Researchers are hoping to determine what part of their inherited genetic make-up makes them develop cancer and what prevents them from recovering from the disease.[5]

If all of them respond the same way, then it must be written in their genetic material to develop cancer, right? Absolutely and 100% yes. Then, why do they need the "cancer-causing agent?" Notice that even though they have the highest genetic predisposition to contracting cancer, they still require the toxin to be introduced into their bodies to develop the cancerous tumors. The genetic program needs to be activated for the body to grow the tumors. Based on this fact, and extensive research performed by Dr. Bruce Lipton, it must be true that genes alone do not cause cancer. The gene for cancer must be turned on or activated in order for cancer to develop. An environmental toxin must be present and when combined with genetic predisposition it will result in the development of cancer. Please recall the discussion on why half the people who smoke heavily never get cancer.

So now, let me answer your question of why do people with a family gene for cancer often develop cancer. Very simply put, it must be because they also get exposed to the same toxins as their relatives from whom they inherited the cancer gene. I'm not saying that their relatives poisoned them. I just believe the gene alone was not enough to cause the cancer. An environmental toxin must have activated the gene at some point in their life.

I wonder how many of the lab mice at the National Cancer Institute would have developed cancer if they hadn't been inbred, genetically altered, and exposed to cancer-causing toxins. Their website reports that in order for them to study the genetic response of these mice, some of them are injected with cancer cells, others are exposed to high doses of radiation, and yet others are given harmful substances like asbestos. So, they poison the mice and then study their genetic response. I fail to see how studying the genetic makeup of the mice will give us any insight into stopping the cancer epidemic. Sounds to me like genes aren't the problem.

When expressing our genetic blueprint the most important factor is our environment. People who may be born with a predisposition for cancer may likely mimic environmental factors of their family such as what they eat and where they live, as well as learned behaviors involving how they handle stress. You should then find great hope and delight in the fact that these environmental triggers are changeable and can be managed.

Dr. Lipton has written books and given hundreds of lectures on this very concept, that the key factor in our health is not our genes, but our environment. How we grow up, what we believe, what we eat, how we handle stress, even how we feel about ourselves, all play a role in our ultimate expression of our genetic health. All of these elements are things we are not born with, but patterns, habits, and beliefs that we develop.

A weak foundation for health is not the result of bad genes it is the result of making bad choices. Illness and poor health are due to toxins and deficiencies in our body. These are outside forces that can be controlled by us. This is great news because it means that if our genes do not determine our health, we can do something about it.

Dr. Lipton further explains that a living cell cannot be in defense and growth at the same time. That means if the body is busy defending against a threat it cannot be growing and thriving. The cells in our body will either move towards growth and health or retreat toward defense and death. In response to its environment, a cell will either express genes that promote repair and regeneration or it will express genes that promote inflammation and illness. When we feed our body toxins, or don't supply the essential nutrients that it needs, we are literally changing our body's genetic expression. Then does it seem logical to wait for illness to appear before we change our environment? The difference is between reacting to disease as opposed to preventing it on a genetic level.

Our healthcare system is focused more on reacting to illness than preventing it. We spend more energy, time and money fixing problems after they occur instead of preventing them from occurring in the first place. If we focused on eating right, moving well, and thinking properly we would improve our health by leaps and bounds.

Even if you are experiencing an illness right now, knowing these facts can help you tap into the healing potential that the innate power in your body wants to express. Understanding the importance of maintaining a friendly environment inside and outside of the body is the key to StressProofing your body and improving your quality of life.

Dr. James Chestnut, author and renowned lecturer, says that "We can only be as healthy as the environment that we live in." When we present with symptoms such as running a fever, vomiting, diarrhea, or something more serious, instead of searching for a way to suppress the symptom, we should consider environmental factors that caused this symptom in the first place. Then we need to take the steps to create a better environment; one that does not oppose the body's innate intelligence but is conducive to healthy genetic expression.

Your future health is the result of the choices you make today. Dr. Chestnut phrases it like this, "your health is determined by how you eat, move and think". The only reason we ever get sick is the same reason we can get well, and that is based on our lifestyle and environmental choices.

Let's end this chapter with an excerpt from Dr. James Chestnut spoken during an interview. His statement here summarizes the function of our genes, the role of innate intelligence, and the effect the environment has on our health.

> "What symptoms do and what symptoms are is a message from the body to the mind to let us know that we need to change our behavior. We need to change our environment. That's why symptoms are so powerful. It's not a mistake to adapt, it's a message to adapt.... raising your blood pressure and cholesterol levels are very intelligent and appropriate for living in a stressful environment, but they can ultimately cause harm if you don't change the environment. Our body, since it has innate intelligence, is always adapting to provide us the best possible chance of survival in any environment, and it always does that to buy us survival time. The fight or flight response isn't about getting us well, it's about giving us time so we can change our environment so we can get well." [6]

Sources:

1. Lenz, Widukind, Dr. "History of Thalidomide." - *Thalidomide*. Association Canadienne Des Victimes De La Thalidomide, 2014. Web

2. Thalidomide: MedlinePlus Drug Information." *U.S National Library of Medicine*. U.S. National Library of Medicine, 25 June 2014. Web

3. Huxley, Rachel R. "Nausea And Vomiting In Early Pregnancy: Its Role In Placenta...: Obstetrics & Gynecology." *Nausea And Vomiting In Early Pregnancy: Its Role In Placenta...: Obstetrics & Gynecology*. American College of Obstetrics & Gynecology, May 2000. Web

4. http://www.nytimes.com/2013/04/16/science/the-human-genome-project-then-and-now.html?_r=0  A version of this interview appeared in print on April 16, 2013, on page D3 of the New York edition with the headline: Human Genome, Then and Now.

5. http://emice.nci.nih.gov/aam/mouse/carcinogen-induced-and-spontaneous-mouse-models

6. Episode 166 SpinalColumnRadio Dr. Thmoas R.  Lamar interview with Dr.James Chestnut

# Chapter 3
# *The Beauty of the Brain and the Nervous System*

*"I am a brain, Watson. The rest of me is a mere appendix."*

- Arthur Conan Doyle, *The Adventure of the Mazarin Stone (one of 12 Sherlock Holmes short stories)*

"5-Foot-3 Woman Lifts Car Off Child" was a headline on the front page of the Spokane Daily Chronicle on December 6, 1979. "I don't know how I did it. My body hurts all over now," said 44-year-old Martha Weiss.[1] How could someone that small conjure so much strength? She didn't even have time to warmup or stretch in preparation. In an instant she became super woman. The article said that she only weighed 118 pounds. Yet, she was able to do something that during normal circumstances she would not be able to do. How did she do it? We will discuss that a bit later in this chapter.

We are moving right along on the path to discovering how to StressProof our life. First we learned that stress is merely a force that causes change in your life. Then we found that our genes do not determine our physiologic destiny and they merely respond and react to an environment filled with various types of stress. Now, we need to discuss the interface between the outside environment and the DNA which is our blueprint of life. If our DNA is isolated in the nucleus at the center of each of our cells, then how does it know what's going on outside of the human body?

Take a look at how the body works. If you wanted to move your index finger, how would you do it? "I would just do it" is probably your response. Well how come the other fingers in your hand don't move? Why doesn't the index finger in the other hand move? What gives you control over your hands and fingers? I just asked my 5 year-old son that very question with multiple choice answers. The choices were the heart, the belly, the head, and the finger moves all by itself. He answered "it's my brain, in my head."

Has your hand ever fallen asleep? For example, at night, have you woken up to find that one of your hands is completely numb? Do you still have full control of your fingers at that moment? If you are a master piano player, would you be able to play the piano at that moment? What do you think caused this temporary loss of function? Is it similar to someone who is paralyzed and confined to a wheelchair and cannot use or control their limbs? If you are thinking about spinal cord trauma, you're on the right track.

Nerves relay information from the brain to the various parts of the body. Your brain tells your finger to move and that information travels along the path of a nerve all the way from the brain to your finger and then and only then the finger moves. If that nerve is no longer connected to your finger, the finger will not move. The brain may keep telling your finger to move but if the nerve signal doesn't reach the muscles that move your finger, the finger will never move.

So then, how does the brain know that it has accomplished its mission of moving the index finger? Is it because your eyes saw your finger move? Try moving your index finger again but this time, close your eyes. You should have noticed that you felt the finger move. You didn't need to see it move to know that it moved. The brain received feedback from the targeted body part, in this case the index finger, informing the brain that the task was accomplished. The same applies to every joint in your body. You don't have to look down at your knees to know if they are bent or straight. Taking this a step further, you don't need to look at yourself in the mirror to know if you're wearing long pants, shorts, or a skirt. You know if it's warm or cold, dark or light, or wet or dry outside, and all of this information travels through neural pathways from the outside environment to the brain. So not only is the brain a command center that controls your actions, it is also a receiving station that monitors and surveys the outside environment.

Then, is the brain the most important and vital part of your body? Or is the heart the most vital part? The heart functions to circulate oxygen-rich blood throughout the body. If we used a machine to pump the blood through the blood vessels we would be able to keep the body alive without a heart. What about the lungs? Again, we can use a machine to force air in and out of the lungs or artificially oxygenate the blood to keep the body alive. Advancements in surgical procedures actually enable us to have heart and lung transplants. That means, a surgeon can replace someone's heart or lungs with those of an organ donor and successfully save a life. It's incredible what a surgeon can do. The same can be done with kidneys and the liver.

Is there an organ in the body that can never be transplanted? Is there an organ in the body that is more vital to life than all other organs? Is there an organ in the body that sustains life and controls all other organs in the body? Yes, you guessed correctly, it's the brain.

When I was in chiropractic school, one of my classes was Gross Anatomy. For four continuous trimesters, during the first two years of the program, I dissected the entire human body for several hours each week. I had to identify every organ, muscle, bone, tissue and gland. I had to trace every blood vessel, artery and vein, back to the heart and I had to trace every nerve back to the spine. I discovered that there is a nerve that goes to every tissue, gland, and organ in the human body and all those nerves are connected to the brain. Why is the brain connected to all other body parts? The answer: in order to control all the functions of the body.

Earlier we defined health as "perfect and proper function and not just the absence of symptoms and disease." Since the brain controls all of the functions of the body, then the brain must be directly responsible for how healthy we are.

If I disconnect the brain from my index finger, will I still be able to move that finger? Is that just a theory, or is that a fact? If I damage the nerves to my right arm, will I still have full use of my right arm? Of course not. Not only will I lose the ability to move my arm, I will also lose the ability to sense and feel with my fingers. Your limbs are in constant and continuous contact with your brain. There are nerve signals that repeatedly travel from your extremities to your brain, constantly reminding your brain of the status of the joints. These are called sensory nerves. Sight, sound, touch, taste, smell, and joint position are all examples of information that regularly travel from the outside world to the brain through sensory nerves. If the nerve signals from one of the legs stops reaching the brain, we say that the leg has "fallen asleep." This sensation can be replicated by sitting on one end of the couch with your legs dangling over the arm rest for an excessively extended period of time (don't try this!). After a few minutes one or both of the legs will fall asleep. At that point the leg is numb and if you try to walk, you won't be able to feel the floor. It will feel like you're walking on stilts. This is all because the compression of the nerves from your leg has blocked all communication between your leg and your brain. This information helps you balance yourself when walking and if it is interrupted, you will easily lose your balance and fall.

The minute your brain realizes that it hasn't heard anything from one of your legs, it starts to search for the leg. The brain could be likened to an overprotective mother who always needs to know where all her children are. Since no information is reaching the brain from the leg, the brain will make that leg hyper-sensitive. Meaning that the leg becomes overly sensitive to any stimulation and at that moment, light touch actually feels like pins and needles. Movement of the leg also causes tingling and in fact the leg may be so sensitive that it actually becomes uncomfortable to move the leg. However, if you shake the leg and stimulate the nerves, the sensitivity will normalize and your leg will begin to feel normal again. Shaking the leg sends a burst of neurologic input to the brain, letting it know that the leg is intact and communication has been reestablished. At that moment the hypersensitivity and pins-and-needles will go away, your balance will be restored and you will have complete control of your leg again.

It is easy to see the relationship between nerves and voluntary movement, but that's not the only thing your brain controls through nerves. Did you know that your brain controls the flow of blood throughout your body? Think about a moment when you were seriously embarrassed. Like having toilet paper stuck to your shoe, or waving at someone you thought you knew but it turned out to be a stranger. The minute you get embarrassed, your face will flush and if your skin isn't too tan you will "turn red." What causes the face to flush or turn red? The answer is increased blood flow. When your mind perceives something as embarrassing, it sends a signal through a specific set of nerves to the skin of the face. The brain tells the small blood vessels (capillaries) of the face to dilate and increase blood flow to the face, in turn causing the face to appear flushed. You see, the face itself doesn't get embarrassed. Information travels to the brain through your sensory nerves such as sight and sound, and the brain interprets that information as embarrassing. Then, it responds by sending signals to the capillaries of your face.

Consider another example of how the brain controls blood vessels and circulation. Remember a moment in life when you were scared for your life. Like a near-miss car accident that could've been disastrous. Chances are, if you were really scared, your face turned pale white, reminiscent of the expression "you look like you've just seen a ghost." The mechanism is the same. Your eyes sent the sensory information to your brain and your brain quickly interpreted the situation as dangerous. At that moment, it sent signals to several body parts to prepare for the potential disaster. By constricting certain blood vessels and dilating others, it took blood from your skin and sent it to your muscles in order to prepare them for fast action. When the blood leaves your face, you turn pale. The signals from the brain also tell your eyes to dilate so that you can let in more light and see your surroundings differently. This process is called the sympathetic response to stress. It is also known as the "fight or flight" response. This physiologic response is what enabled our 5-foot-3 Martha Weiss to be able to lift a car off of the child. We will discuss this response by the nervous system in more detail later in this chapter. For now, what's important to understand is that even the flow of blood is under the direct control of the brain and nervous system.

While the brain's control of muscles and joints is voluntary, the brain's control of blood flow is involuntary. In other words, you can easily decide when and how to move the index finger but you more than likely cannot increase the flow of blood toward your left kidney. Can you make your heart stop beating right now? Can you make it stop beating even for just a minute? Yet, your heart actually knows when it should beat faster and when it should slow down.

How does it know these things? The answer is that your heart and many of your other organs and glands are under the control of the autonomic nervous system. This is the section of the brain that automatically controls essential functions of the body that keep you alive. The good news is that you will never accidentally forget to make your heart beat. It is automatically controlled by your brain without the requirement of conscious thought. In fact when you think of the autonomic nervous system, just think of the word automatic.

Earlier in this chapter we discussed the sympathetic response to stress which is more commonly referred to as the "fight or flight" response. It is the response that allowed the woman in our story to lift a car when needed. This is one of those automatic functions. In fact the autonomic nervous system serves two purposes in the body. One is called the sympathetic response and the other is called the parasympathetic response. This system can be likened to a car that has a gas pedal and a brake pedal. The sympathetic nervous system is like the gas pedal and is used to speed up certain functions like heart rate and metabolism. The parasympathetic system, more commonly referred to as the "rest and digest" response, is used to slow down those same functions.

As we discussed earlier, the sympathetic nervous system gets activated during times of danger - like when a car is on top of a child. When the sympathetic nervous system is activated, the adrenal glands will release adrenaline, the heart will beat faster, and breathing intensifies. The pupils of the eyes dilate to let in more light. This is when blood is drawn away from the skin and certain internal organs such as the stomach and the intestines. Most of the blood is directed by the nervous system to supply the muscles with oxygen and food. In this instance digestion completely stops and the body is prepared to take actions related to "fight or flight." When I was on the track team in high school, I regularly saw our elite athletes throw up right before the big race. The reason was that they were in "fight or flight" and digestion had seized. Therefore their body had to get rid of their stomach contents.

The opposite of the sympathetic nervous system is the parasympathetic nervous system. The parasympathetic system is activated when there is no perceived danger. Imagine that you just ate a large and delicious meal that you thoroughly enjoyed. Now you are lounging on the couch, your legs are outstretched with your feet on the coffee table. You are so relaxed that you are about to doze off into a deep peaceful sleep. This is the parasympathetic response and that is why it is commonly referred to as the "rest and digest" or "wine and dine" response. In this instance, most of the blood flow is directed toward the intestines and the stomach to promote digestion. The more relaxed you are the better your body can digest the food and use the nutrients to supply the rest of your body. All healing, repair, and regeneration of tissues, organs, and glands occur under the control of the parasympathetic nervous system. The parasympathetic nervous system is also hard at work when we are sleeping.

All of this occurs automatically and is not under your voluntary control, and, while that is true, you do have a degree of influence on the overall autonomic responses of your body. For example, you can actually activate your parasympathetic system by eating a large meal, doing a breathing exercise, meditating, or sleeping. You can also activate your sympathetic response by worrying, watching a horror movie, gambling, or taking a polar plunge in arctic waters. When we worry, the body responds in the same way as when something bad actually happens. The emotions of worry, fear, anger, and anxiety can activate the sympathetic response, while emotions of love, joy, gratitude, and hope will most likely stimulate a parasympathetic response. Since all healing, repair, and regeneration occur in the parasympathetic state, which emotions would you rather experience more often?

In the last chapter we talked about Dr. Lipton's work and his conclusion that a cell cannot be in growth and defense at the same time. Similarly, the body cannot be in a sympathetic and parasympathetic state at the same time. This would be like pressing the gas pedal and the brake pedal of a car at the same time. The car wouldn't know what to do. The engine would rev, the car would jerk, but it wouldn't actually go anywhere. In the same way, you cannot sleep if you are in sympathetic overdrive. That would be like relaxing into a deep comfortable sleep while being chased by a pack of hungry wolves. The instant the wolves appear, you will enter a state of heightened awareness. You will be more alert than if you had just consumed a hundred cups of coffee (don't try this!).

Both the sympathetic and parasympathetic systems are necessary for survival and there needs to be balance between the two systems. An imbalance between the two can be very detrimental to health. Unfortunately, in today's fast-paced world, many people are living their life in sympathetic dominance. Over the past 24 hours, if you worried about money or paying your bills, you activated the sympathetic system. If you had an argument with a family member or coworker, you activated the sympathetic nervous system. If you got stuck in traffic, were late for work, got yelled at by your boss, missed a deadline, or received bad news, you are most likely in sympathetic overdrive. Simply watching the news can send you into sympathetic overdrive.

Normally it wouldn't be a problem to have a "fight or flight" response to an event, especially if it helps you lift a car off of a child, as long as the body has time to balance itself with time spent in a parasympathetic state of "rest and digest." Unfortunately, many of us in America don't even take time to sit down and enjoy a nice lunch. Instead, we eat on the go, in our car, or at our desk while working on the computer. How can the body attempt to "rest and digest" if the person is always in a state of heightened awareness? If the body has no time to heal, repair and regenerate in the "rest and digest" parasympathetic state, it will begin to breakdown and decay. The body was not designed to remain in sympathetic overdrive long-term.

Do not mistakenly link the state of sympathetic overdrive with feeling emotional stress. Even if you are not emotionally experiencing a lot of stress, the act of not resting or relaxing can be severely detrimental to your health. This thought makes me think of technology greats like Steve Jobs. Throughout the years of his stellar career he regularly put in long continuous hours of work without much rest. He may not have been feeling stress from this and in fact, he probably reported that he enjoyed his work. Meanwhile, he was not allowing time for his body to rest and repair.

Even when you do not feel stress, you may be in a state of sympathetic overdrive. Today, there are many young professionals striving for success in their field and they're filling their bodies with unhealthy stimulants and energy drinks so that they can stay alert and productive through long workdays. This behavior keeps their bodies in sympathetic overdrive. Their bodies will not last because they are not allowing enough time for the parasympathetic nervous system to activate the processes of healing, repair, and regeneration.

The exact opposite of this is the "French Paradox." In France the incidence of heart disease is very low when compared to other western nations. However, their intake of saturated fats and cholesterol-rich foods is very high.[2] Hence the paradox that if their diet is so bad, then why don't they have more heart attacks? I believe the answer lies in the French culture and their attitude toward food and eating. As an American vacationing in France, I couldn't help but notice how much longer they spend at the dining table during mealtime. Our dinners would last at least two hours.

In the U.S. it is common to tell your restaurant server that you are in a hurry and ask them to bring your check when the food comes out. Such behavior in France would be misconstrued as disrespect for the food, the chef, and the restaurant. So, as it is their culture, the French typically sit down and relax when they eat, and they take their time, eating slowly and savoring every bite. Which side of the nervous system do you think this behavior will activate? If you said "wine and dine" or "rest and digest," you are correct. This is the embodiment of the parasympathetic nervous system.

Who do you think will process their food in a healthier fashion; the American couple who is rushing through their meal because they're worried about missing the show or the start of the play? Or the French couple who is calmly enjoying their meal and in no rush to leave the restaurant?

Food is intended to stimulate the parasympathetic response which in turn promotes proper digestion, strengthens the immune system, slows the heartrate, decreases blood pressure, and creates an environment in your body that is ideal for rest, repair, and regeneration. When we eat on the go, rushed and nervous, we stay in sympathetic overdrive and never really process our food properly. So in conclusion, how we eat is just as important as and perhaps even more important than what we eat. The person who eats super healthy foods but rushes through his meal is more likely to have a heart attack than the person who may not eat as healthy but maintains a peaceful state of mind while eating.

My patient, Lauren, is an eighth grade school teacher for the public school system. Her chief complaint was that once or twice a week, she woke up with a stiff neck and had trouble turning her head. Anti-inflammatories and pain medications were helpful but the stiffness always returned a few days later. As we spoke about her condition, I realized that she had a long list of symptoms that she had assumed were unrelated to her stiff neck. Some of the symptoms she complained about included:

- Her hands and feet were always cold
- High blood pressure
- High cholesterol
- Indigestion
- Acid reflux
- Constipation
- Insomnia
- Frequent head colds
- Frequent sinus infections
- And an inability to lose her ever-increasing belly fat

She was undergoing care with a number of specialists which included:

- A cardiologist who prescribed medication for high blood pressure and high cholesterol
- A gastroenterologist who suggested over-the-counter antacids and stool softeners
- A primary care physician who prescribed a low dose sedative for insomnia and recommended that she continue to take Ibuprofen for her recurrent neck pain

She was also advised that she was pre-diabetic and if she didn't lose weight she would wind up with diabetes.

She considered herself healthy because she believed that the medications were "making" her healthy.

So I asked her how she handled stress in her life.

As a junior high school teacher she dealt with pre-teens, young teenagers, and their "crazy hormones." The parents of her students regularly blamed her for their child's lack of effort and poor grades. She was also experiencing an enormous amount of stress from the school administration that constantly changed the curriculum. As well, she had to spend her spare time devoted to responsibilities related to her job for which she was underpaid.

From the details of her life, it is pretty obvious that Lauren was stuck in sympathetic overdrive. Her body was in a constant state of "fight or flight." Although her team of physicians had separated her different symptoms into distinct categories, I felt certain that they were all related. So let's break it down.

The first sign of sympathetic activation is increased heart rate which causes high blood pressure. When the state of "fight or flight" persists or recurs too frequently, cortisol levels will increase. Cortisol is commonly known as the stress hormone. It is produced by the adrenal glands; the same glands that produce adrenalin during stressful times. While adrenaline may help you lift a car, cortisol helps the body use sugar and fat as energy. It mobilizes triglycerides and cholesterol in the blood. Triglycerides and cholesterol are precursors to other very important hormones such as estrogen and testosterone. This is why someone who has elevated blood pressure as a result of chronic sympathetic overdrive, will also have elevated serum cholesterol levels.

So, why are her hands cold all the time, even during the summer? Recall that when faced with a dangerous situation that elicits a "fight or flight" response, the body will constrict blood vessels in the skin and the extremities (hands and feet) in order to direct that blood to the muscles in preparation for emergency action. If she is in chronic sympathetic overdrive, her hands and feet will naturally have poor circulation which renders them constantly cold.

Also recall that during the "fight or flight" response, the body stops all digestive activities in order to direct the blood and other resources to the muscles. When being chased by the proverbial saber-tooth tiger, the brain isn't worried about whether you're digesting your food. No wonder she had indigestion and constipation. Her body is always preparing for a fight and isn't taking enough time to focus on "rest and digest."

This is the same reason she gets frequent head colds and sinus infections, because, the resources of the body are too often being taken away from the immune system and directing their attention to supplying the large muscles with what they need to escape the proverbial saber-tooth tiger and lift the car off of the child. Chronic sympathetic overdrive significantly weakens the immune system.

How is all this related to her pre-diabetic status? I mentioned earlier that cortisol increases blood sugar levels because sugar is the fuel that sustains muscle activity. However, elevated blood sugar levels sustained over a long period of time will eventually result in diabetes. Incidentally to maintain such high energy states of blood sugar and cholesterol, cortisol tends to increase appetite and odd cravings. As a result people in this type of chronic sympathetic overdrive tend to gain excessive belly fat which is nearly impossible to lose if the patient stays in the state of "fight or flight."

It may sound like I'm blaming everything on the hormone cortisol. That's not the case. Cortisol is very beneficial to the body and in a normal individual it fluctuates in a cyclical manner throughout the 24 hour circadian cycle. However, when it is excessively released without giving the body a chance to recover, it will result in:

- Blood sugar imbalance
- Decreased bone density and osteoporosis
- Sleep disruption
- Decreased muscle mass
- Elevated blood pressure
- Lowered immune function
- Increased abdominal fat
- Increased inflammation in the body

It is that last item on the above list that explains the recurring neck pain and stiffness. Recall that she said the over-the-counter anti-inflammatories help her feel better but the pain keeps coming back.

An individual who is under constant negative emotional stress and has trouble sleeping at night probably has a tendency to be very tense in her neck and shoulders. The whole thing is the perfect storm and a recipe for disaster. Her problem is not a musculoskeletal issue. It is not a gastrointestinal issue. It certainly is not a cardiovascular issue. This is a nervous system issue.

The story had a happy ending. I was able to restore balance between her sympathetic and parasympathetic nervous systems and once this was established, her symptoms began to disappear. She gradually went off all medication and even began to lose weight. All of this was accomplished through chiropractic care of the spine and the "Simple Seven" which you will read about in the next two chapters.

Notice that we have spent a lot of time discussing sympathetic overdrive and not a whole lot of discussion regarding parasympathetic dominance. The reason is that in today's culture parasympathetic over-dominance is not too prevalent. However, to be fair, let's spend just a few minutes on that right now.

Parasympathetic overdrive can also result in negative symptoms. Those may include increased salivation, abnormally low blood pressure, increased mucous production, bronchial constriction that can cause wheezing in the lungs, being overly emotional, and increased/frequent urination. This is exactly why autonomic balance is so important to our health.

So thus far we've discussed three divisions of the nervous system and provided a general overview of their function.

Here is a quick recap of those systems:

1. The sensory nervous system – brings information from the outside environment to the brain. This includes:

    a. Vision
    b. Hearing
    c. Smell
    d. Taste
    e. Touch
    f. Temperature
    g. Sense of joint position
    h. Pain

2. Voluntary nervous system – sends information outward from the brain to the parts of the body that you have complete control over, i.e. the musculoskeletal system. It's functions include:

    a. Movement
    b. Balance
    c. Coordination
    d. Chewing
    e. Swallowing (this one also happens automatically)

3. Autonomic nervous system – automatically controls the involuntary functions of the body. Included are:

    a. Organs such as the heart, lungs, stomach, intestines, kidneys, liver, spleen and pancreas. Their functions include:

        • Heart rate
        • Respiration rate
        • Digestion
        • Metabolism

   b.  Glands such as salivary glands, tear glands, and sweat glands. Their functions include:

- Saliva production
- Tear production
- Sweating

   c.  Blood vessels. Autonomic control of the blood vessels allow for:

- Blood flow to the stomach and intestines during digestion
- Blood flow to the muscles and joints during exercise

Keep in mind that for the purposes of this book I'm not planning to discuss the higher functions of the human brain such as cognition and memory which mostly occur in the cerebral cortex and the limbic system of the brain. These higher functions of the brain include conscious thought, special reasoning, and language. The limbic system of the brain controls functions such as emotion, behavior, motivation, long term memory and learning.

So the brain controls all functions of the body. The spinal cord is the information highway that allows for the transmission of information from the brain to the body parts and from the environment back to the brain. This explains why damage to the spinal cord can be so detrimental to the body.

On May 27, 1995, Christopher Reeve was thrown from a horse during an equestrian competition in Virginia. The fall caused irreparable damage to his spinal cord and as a result, he was confined to a wheelchair, required a breathing apparatus, and needed assistance with bowel and bladder functions for the rest of his life. Prior to his injury Mr. Reeve was an actor, famous for his role as the iconic Superman. Why is it that after his injury, Superman could no longer move his arms and legs, and lost other bodily functions including his ability to breathe? Did he damage his lungs in the fall? No. Did he injure his arms and legs? No. His injury was to the neck. If the brain controls all of those functions and the injury occurred below the brain, in the spinal cord, then why did he lose so many functions? The answer is that the vital information from the brain was no longer able to travel down the spinal cord into his organs, his arms, and his legs. It is obvious that the spinal cord is just as important as the brain when it comes to the health and function of the body. Neither one can sustain life without the other.

Here's where it all becomes very interesting. Visualize for an instant that you are in front of the New York Philharmonic, witnessing a masterful display of musical talent from the musicians who beautifully accompany each other in tone, pitch, rhythm, and volume. The result is breathtaking. So what's with the guy wearing the long tail tuxedo standing up front waving the stick at the musicians? He's not making any musical sounds, right? Why is he there? Dumb question! He's the conductor. The orchestra can't do without him. So what would happen if one of the musicians had an obstructed view and couldn't see the conductor? He or she may not be able to keep up with the rest of the orchestra and this musician may even ruin the sound of the entire band. In this scenario, does it mean that this poor musician suddenly lost her musical talent, or did this happen because of the obstruction blocking her view of the conductor? The obstruction in this scenario is the same as the spinal cord injury that Christopher Reeve suffered.

So exchange the conductor with the brain, and exchange the musicians with the organs, glands, blood vessels, and muscles. You see, your brain is currently and always, doing what the conductor of the orchestra was doing. It is sending information out to the various tissues of the body to ensure that your body continues to play the proverbial beautiful music. If there is ever an obstruction in the system of nerves, such as a spinal cord injury, the brain (conductor) would not be able to get the message out to a certain organ (musician). The consequence of this would be disastrous. What if this obstruction has affected communication between the brain and the heart? Will the heart continue to function the way the brain wants it to? In this case there is nothing wrong with the heart itself, and there's certainly nothing wrong with the brain but there is miscommunication between the brain and the heart, causing the heart to have trouble keeping up with the rest of the musicians. Intervention is necessary. The question is, what type of intervention should we use? Should it be in the form of chemicals that bypass the nervous system and artificially control the heart? Or should it be focused on restoring communication between the brain and the heart?

Let's explore that more in the next chapter.

By now you should have a whole new understanding of the concept of stress, genetics, and the nervous system.

In the first chapter we discussed that stress is a force that causes change in your life. It is not stress itself but the body's ability to adapt to stress that determines how healthy you are. To achieve true wellness you need to improve all three dimensions of health (physical, chemical and psychological) simultaneously.

In the second chapter, I explained that genes don't determine your health. Your genetics provide you with options to respond to your environment and it's really the environment that determines how your genes express themselves. Furthermore, we discussed the role of innate intelligence in the body. It is the wisdom of the body that knows exactly when and how to respond to its environment in order to increase your chances of survival.

And in this chapter, we talked about the importance of the brain and nervous system. The nervous system is the interface between the environment on the outside and the DNA or genes on the inside. It is of vital importance that the brain is able to receive accurate information about the outside environment and in turn be able to send out or relay instructional information to the various components of the body. The mental impulse received by the target organ will activate the appropriate genetic program that enables that organ to respond accordingly. Activation of the wrong genetic program will cause disease and illness. Activation of the right genetic program will cause health and wellness. Any obstruction or interference in this system of communication will render the body unable to appropriately respond to stress.

In the next chapter, I'm going to discuss how to remove the interference to ensure optimal function.

Sources:

1. Spokane Daily Chronicle 94th Year. No. 66. Spokane, Wash., Thursday, Dec. 6, 1979.

2. Jean Ferrières, The French paradox: Lessons for other countries, Heart. 2004 Jan; 90(1): 107–111

# Chapter 4
## *Get Adjusted*

*"The doctor of the future will give no medicine but will interest his patients in the care of the human frame, in diet, and in the cause and prevention of disease."*

- Thomas Edison

## Dr. Kevin's Story:

*When I was four years old Medical specialists told my parents that I was permanently brain damaged. I've been arguing with these so called specialists ever since.*

*Shortly after being born I started throwing febrile seizures, my body temperature would rise and when it spiked, I would go into convulsions. At first the doctors thought that the seizures were caused by an infection so they prescribed high doses of antibiotics. The antibiotics didn't help but my parents reluctantly followed the doctors' advice changing and filling one prescription after another. My mother disliked the idea of drugging her infant son but hated witnessing the seizures even more. She begged the doctors to try something other than antibiotics. The Doctors reasoned that since my seizures always followed a fever, all my mother had to do was to keep my body temperature down with high doses of Tylenol and ice baths.*

*My mother was so tired of feeding me drugs that she opted for the ice baths. When my temperature started to rise she would run to the freezer and grab all the ice and empty it in the bath tub, run cold water and hold me in the tub of freezing water until the temperature subsided. She said it was awful, I would be kicking and screaming but she would pin me down and hold me in the tub for as long as it took. At first, this technique would shock my central nervous system enough to impede the convulsions, but the frequency of the fevers increased over time. My poor mother. Sometimes my fever would spike before the water in her ice trays refroze. She was so determined that the ice baths were going to cure the seizures that she would grab me under her arms and run through the neighborhood screaming at the top of her voice that she needed ice. The neighbors thought she was nuts but one lady would always open her door, empty all of her ice in her bath tub and help my mother pin me down until the fever subsided.*

*As I got older, the seizures worsened and they were having a harder and harder time holding me down in the ice baths. There was only so much kicking and screaming that they could take. That is when they demanded to see some more specialists. The first specialist said that I must have meningitis and the only way to test for that was by doing a spinal tap. They informed my Father that he would have to hold me in the fetal-position while they withdrew some cerebrospinal fluid from my spine. My dad is a tough looking cowboy, and at the time he was also the coach of the high school football team, so the doctors thought he would be able to hold me down just fine. The thing with most tough looking guys is that they are soft as hell in the inside. My mother said that as soon as they brought the needle out to perform the spinal tap, the kicking and screaming began. It turns out dad has a terrible fear of needles, he was crying his heart out as he held his son in the fetal position while the specialist jammed a six inch needle into my spine.*

*The spinal tap came back negative for meningitis, but the specialists decided to give me the meningococcal antibiotic anyway. My father was infuriated, why did they have to perform a spinal tap if they were just going to prescribe the same drugs regardless of the lab results? What kind of risks were they taking by sticking a needle into the spine of a child? What the hell is wrong with these so called specialists?*

*The antibiotic didn't help, and six months later we are at a new specialist's office. These doctors convinced my parents to perform an electroencephalogram to measure brain wave activity. They had instructed my parents to* shave all the hair off of my head and to be prepared to help out. This was the mid 1970's and medical technology wasn't near what it is today. The nurses rolled in a strange looking machine with a dozen or so wires hanging from it and asked my father to help them hold me down. He wasn't sure what to expect and nearly lost his mind when they started plunging the bare wire leads deep into my skull. I was four years old at this time and although I don't have much recollection of any of my childhood I remember that test, it hurt like hell! I was kicking and screaming and being held down by my mother while across the room, my dad was kicking and screaming and being held down by the nurses.

The electroencephalogram test results came back positive, in a very negative way. The specialists sat my parents down and told them that I had epilepsy and permanent brain damage. They explained that parts of my brain were not functioning and that I would never be able to read or write, play sports or attend a "normal" school. They said that the epilepsy could be treated with more drugs but that a seizure could occur at any time, they recommended that I wear a helmet anytime that I was outside.

My parents left this appointment completely devastated. They drove to the pharmacy and filled the prescriptions of Phenobarbital, Dilantin, and even more antibiotics. They then drove to a sport store and got me fitted for a stupid white helmet. As mentioned earlier I don't remember much about my childhood but I remember that stupid white helmet, I hated that damn thing!

I was five years old, and again it was the mid 1970's, nobody wore helmets back then. I would go outside to play road hockey with my older brother and the neighborhood kids and I was the only one wearing a helmet. Even the *goalie would be in net with a couple phone books taped to his shins, but no helmet. The taunts of "Hey, helmet-head" and "what's the matter crash-baby" were unyielding. I got so frustrated that I would walk over to the side of the street and pick up all the small rocks and put them in my pockets. When the kids would tease me I would throw the rocks at them and a full out rock fight would ensue!*

*My poor mother was losing her mind! She couldn't let me go outside to play without my helmet because she was terrified that I would have a seizure and crack my head open. But, if I went outside with the helmet on, I would end up throwing rocks at the neighborhood kids and could possibly crack their heads open. She had now been coping with over five years of seizures, drugs, ice baths, spinal taps, electroencephalograms, and now rock fights. She was stressed out and needed help! This is when one of the neighborhood ladies suggested that she go see her chiropractor, Dr. Clark Lundgren.*

*Dr. Lundgren practiced in a town 2 hours away, so my mom strapped that stupid white helmet to my head, packed my bag of drugs, and took me along for the ride. She went in to get her adjustment and came out feeling great. As she was packing me up to leave Dr. Lundgren came out and asked "Irene, does your son throw seizures?" She answered "yes, how did you know that?" He said that he noticed that my ear was much lower on one side than the other, and that one eye was drooping. He went on to explain that if the skull doesn't sit properly on top of the spine the central nervous system can be stressed and seizures will manifest. He then asked my mother about my birth. She reported that the birth had been awful and that the doctors had rushed the delivery using a great deal of force with forceps. She told him that the entire right side of my face had been swollen and my right eye was black and blue from the trauma of being born.*

*Dr. Lundgren asked my mother if he could examine me and when she said yes, he immediately took me in and ran a simple x-ray of my neck and skull. He developed the x-rays and sat my mother down to show her what he had found. The traumatic birth had dislodged the base of my skull so badly that it was causing interference with the cerebellum and brainstem; he called this a subluxation. The cerebellum and brainstem are the parts of your brain that are responsible for movement, balance, and equilibrium. Disruption of these areas could definitely cause seizures and present as clinical brain damage. My mother was shocked, why hadn't the other specialists figured this out?*

*Dr. Lundgren then asked if he could give me an adjustment to correct the subluxation that was causing a miscommunication between my brain and body. Like I have said, I don't recall anything about my childhood except the electroencephalogram, the stupid white helmet and now, what happened next. Dr. Lundgren asked my mother to hold on to my feet, he leaned over and cradled my head in his hands and as my mom held my feet he performed what is called an Occipital Lift adjustment. I remember this loud "Pop" and my eyes flew open like a shot of electricity had just passed through my body, I could feel blood rushing to my head and I could feel that my power was turned on. I looked over at my mother and her eyes rolled back in her head, she lost her power and she collapsed to the ground. Five years of stress had finally caught up to her and caused her to faint. I remember watching Dr. Lundgren calmly walk around the table, softly slap my mom on the face and tell her that everything was going to be okay. He told her to take me home and throw all the drugs (and that stupid white helmet) in the garbage. I remember leaving the office and my mother looking over her shoulder to make sure Dr. Lundgren didn't see her put the helmet on my head as we went outside. I remember going home and seeing my mom put the bag of drugs in the cabinet over the fridge, "just in case". I also remember mom reading to me a few months after that adjustment and how shocked she was when I started reading back to her. I remember being able to read and do math before starting the first grade of a "normal" school. I also remember excelling at school, playing every possible sport and only wearing helmets when I absolutely had to!*

*Dr. Lundgren's adjustment turned my power on, freed up the full potential of my innate intelligence and has allowed me to live life to the fullest. I am now practicing chiropractic, married to my wife who is a Chiropractor, and owe my life to ChiropracTIC.*

The above is the real-life story of Dr. Kevin Watson, written in his own words. Together with his wife Dr. Marcia Watson, they own and operate a successful chiropractic practice in Edmonton, Alberta, Canada.

## *What Is Chiropractic?*

"You get your back cracked and you feel better," is what the woman sitting next to me on the airplane said, when I asked her what she knew about chiropractic. She followed that statement by saying "Thank goodness I've never needed to see a chiropractor; I've never had back pain." Well, Dr. Kevin didn't have back pain either, but he credits chiropractic with saving his life. Shouldn't we learn a bit more about this thing called chiropractic?

"Get knowledge of the spine, for this is the requisite for many diseases." - Hippocrates, Greek physician and the father of modern medicine (460-370 B.C.)

Chiropractic was discovered in 1895 by Daniel David Palmer. He believed that spinal alignment directly affects the function of the nerves, the spinal cord, and the brain. He built the chiropractic profession on the basis that an abnormality in the spine will interfere with the health of the individual.

Over the past century there have been many published research articles and case studies that support D. D. Palmer's claims. There are also many experts and specialists who dispute Palmer's claims, stating that spinal misalignments cannot affect the function of the spinal cord and cannot interfere with nerve impulse conduction.

The fact is, currently chiropractic is the second largest field in healthcare and the largest of the "alternative to medicine" professions. Incidentally, it is also one of the youngest fields in healthcare. It is newer than acupuncture, homeopathy, naturopathy, osteopathy, and Ayurvedic medicine. Why is it that one of the youngest fields in healthcare has quickly become the most popular and successful among alternatives to mainstream medicine? Would it have grown so much and so fast if it wasn't effective? Would it have so much support and such a strong following if it didn't work?

Since its inception in 1895, chiropractic has passed the test of time. It has been on trial and was upheld by the Supreme Court of the United States in Wilk v. American Medical Association. The literature supports its effectiveness to the point that the United States Government, the Veterans Administration, Medicare, and all major insurance companies will cover and reimburse chiropractic services.

So, what is chiropractic?

Chiropractic is the method by which the health of the spine is analyzed and enhanced. The spine protects the spinal cord and supports your body weight. That alone is enough reason to make spinal health a priority.

Consider the profession of dentistry. It is the method by which the health of your teeth are analyzed and enhanced. The teeth serve to help with digestion and primarily are used to bite, tear, and chew food. Dentists claim that if teeth are not properly maintained, the result will be tooth decay and gum disease. They further claim that if misalignments in teeth are not corrected using braces, they can result in problems with biting, chewing, and speaking as well as headaches and earaches. In fact, most dentists will state that a healthy mouth makes for a healthy body.

I can't think of anyone who would publicly disagree with any of these claims about dentistry. If these claims are true about teeth, then how much more important is it to maintain a healthy spine? If a misalignment of teeth can cause earaches and headaches, how much more can a misaligned spine affect your health?

At a recent business convention, the CEO of a mid-size company told me that he would never go to a chiropractor because "once you have something 'cracked' you have to keep getting it 'cracked' and it'll never feel normal again unless you keep cracking it."

That wasn't the first time I heard that one. It's rarely spoken by people who have experienced an actual chiropractic adjustment. Typically people say this because of a past experience that caused them to fear chiropractic. Or, they may be someone who has a habit of cracking their knuckles. As with any habit, they seem to keep doing it and tend to mistakenly believe that adjusting the spine is similar to cracking their knuckles. This couldn't be further from the truth.

Others attempt to adjust their own necks and backs. This is not advisable because it is impossible to deliver a specific chiropractic adjustment to oneself. You will either fail to correct the specific misalignment or you will move the spinal joints beyond their normal range of motion. Neither scenario is very desirable.

A chiropractic adjustment, by definition, must be specific. For example, through an x-ray analysis, your chiropractor may find that the first bone in your neck, called the Atlas (or C1), is tilted to the left or rotated to the left. Your chiropractor would then contact only the bone or vertebra that is misaligned and apply a very specific force in a very specific direction to return only that vertebra, in this case C1, back to its normal and natural position. Once this adjustment takes place, and assuming there are no other subluxations in your spine, you will most likely lose your ability and desire to "pop your own neck." Also the health benefits of a specific adjustment are endless.

As I explained this to the CEO at the business convention, he asked, "Then why do people have to keep going back to the chiropractor?"

That is a valid question. Most of my patients continue to see me as their chiropractor for many years. They refer their children, siblings, parents, and friends and encourage them to stay under care long term. So, I don't blame you if you also believe that once you see a chiropractor, you're stuck having to go for the rest of your life. However, the premise behind this belief is where the confusion arises.

I respectfully explained to him that just by having a chiropractic adjustment, you don't become dependent on getting regular adjustments. That's like saying once you start exercising in a gym, you have to keep going for the rest of your life. Or, once you start eating organically grown produce, you have to continue doing it for the rest of your life. Similarly, it's like saying once you see a dentist for a professional dental cleaning, you have to keep going for the rest of your life. Or, once you brush your teeth, you have to regularly brush them for the rest of your life. You would laugh if I said, once you have your cholesterol checked, you have to keep getting it checked for the rest of your life. My CEO friend got the point. At the end of our conversation he asked if I could recommend a chiropractor in his area.

The fact is that you may choose to see a chiropractor for a specific period of time in order to correct a spinal problem, or like most people, you may decide that you would like to maintain proper spinal hygiene by visiting your chiropractor regularly on an ongoing basis. The truth is that you don't have to, but why wouldn't you go to a chiropractor regularly for the rest of your life? It's the perfect way to protect your greatest investment, which is your health.

To expand on this point, let's continue the comparison between chiropractic and dentistry. What does a dentist most commonly search for when examining your teeth? Cavities! What does a chiropractor search for when examining your spine? Subluxations! The difference is that a subluxation is a whole lot more serious and detrimental than a cavity. A subluxation is a neuro-spinal dysfunction.

In other words, it is a problem in the spine that affects the function of the spinal cord and spinal nerves. Recall from the previous chapter that nerves are used by the brain to monitor and communicate with all parts of the body including organs, glands, blood vessels, joints, and muscles. Therefore a subluxation is anything that interferes with the brain's ability to properly monitor and control the functions of your organs, glands, blood vessels, joints and muscles.

If you have teeth, you are undeniably susceptible to cavities and if you have a spine, you are most definitely susceptible to subluxations. What would happen if you decided to ignore a tooth cavity and not get it filled by your dentist? The common belief is that the cavity will rot through the entire tooth, painfully irritating the nerve and then begin to affect the surrounding teeth. Eventually, it will cause tooth decay and gum disease in the entire mouth. Comparatively, let's discuss what would happen if you decided to ignore a spinal subluxation and not get an adjustment to correct it. The affected spinal joint will begin to degenerate, become arthritic, and irritate the nerve root. The arthritis will spread to the surrounding vertebral joints and eventually cause arthritis throughout a large region of the spine.

Have you ever gone to a dentist for a routine checkup and been given the bad news that you have a tooth cavity? Why didn't you already know about the cavity? Why did you have to wait until the dentist told you about it? This is because a cavity has no signs or symptoms in its early stages, and by the time the tooth begins to hurt, the cavity is most likely so advanced that the tooth may need a root canal or worse, the tooth may need to be extracted. In the same way, a subluxation by definition is silent or asymptomatic. Meaning, it typically has no signs and symptoms. In fact by the time a subluxation begins to cause pain, it has already advanced to arthritis – inflamed spinal joints and degeneration. So you don't necessarily have to feel anything to have a tooth cavity and you certainly don't have to have any pain to have a subluxation in your spine.

If someone has a tooth cavity can he or she fix the problem by exercising, doing yoga, taking pills, or getting acupuncture? Of course not! All of those things are helpful in their own way but they do not fix or fill a tooth cavity. In the same way, if someone has a misalignment or subluxation in the spine, he or she will not be able to correct the problem by doing yoga, getting a massage, lifting weights, taking vitamins, eating broccoli, medicating, or getting injections.

Thankfully there is a safe and effective way to have our subluxations corrected before and after debilitating consequences set in. And that's the amazing and powerful chiropractic adjustment. Just as a cavity can only be fixed by a dentist, an adjustment can only be delivered by a qualified, trained, licensed, and board certified chiropractor.

So, if you don't necessarily feel subluxations, how can you know if you have one? How does a chiropractor determine if a subluxation is present in your spine? The answer is very similar to how your dentist determines if you have a cavity in your teeth. Your dentist will examine your teeth but to be certain, he or she will routinely take x-rays to look for cavities. A chiropractor will also take x-rays to measure and analyze the alignment of the vertebral column and determine if a subluxation exists.

Although x-rays are most valuable in detecting subluxations, they are not solely sufficient in determining the presence of a subluxation. The chiropractor will also look for neurologic patterns which may have been functionally affected in your body. This is because, by definition, a subluxation must affect the function of the nervous system. Patterns of neurologic dysfunction are determined by the following types of testing: balance and coordination testing, thermal patterns surrounding the spine revealing blood circulation irregularities, and muscle tone analysis at rest and in motion.

If you are like a lot of my patients, your eyes began to glaze over as you read the last sentence. I completely understand that not everyone shares my enthusiasm and passion for the scientific basis in support of subluxations. Therefore, if you would like, you have my permission to skip to subluxations on page 123. However, if you are a science geek like me, then buckle your seat belts because I'm going to take us on a scientific journey to explore the supportive evidence behind subluxation and the efficacy of chiropractic.

Since a misalignment alone is not enough to confidently conclude that there is a problem, we use these subluxation models to determine if the nervous system is being affected and to what extent it is damaging your health.[1]

- *Dyskenesia* – also known as pathomechanics. This refers to abnormal segmental motion in the spinal column. Abnormal motion in a specific segment of the vertebral column will result in ligamentous tugging. Ligaments are tissues that are found around every joint and their job is to hold two bones together. Ligaments are strong fibrous tissues that have almost no elasticity, meaning they do not stretch or elongate under tensile stress. This is why a misalignment will result in tugging of the ligaments around the joint. Tugging of the ligaments and abnormal motion of the segment will result in focal inflammation which can be seen on an MRI. This inflammation in the joint when left uncorrected, will result in degenerative changes and fluid in the marrow of the bones at the areas where the affected ligaments are attached. Again, this is not visible on an x-ray and will be easily missed unless we use a high resolution MRI. Finally, when this condition is left alone, it will result in osteophytosis (formation of bone spurs). The bone density must change between 30 and 50% from normal before the degeneration can be visible on an x-ray. Some experts have said that it may take up to 15 years of degenerative change before a bone spur is large enough and dense enough to be seen on an x-ray. The point here is that a subluxation can go undetected for many years. During that entire time progressive degeneration is taking place and will eventually result in permanent loss of joint function. Furthermore, the resulting disc protrusion, bone spurs, and ligament hypertrophy (thickening) will cause narrowing of the spinal canal which will ultimately cause spinal cord compression. This type of degenerative change will not only cause local irritation and pain but it can also cause compression of the nerve roots which are the major extensions of the spinal cord that branch off to exit the spinal column and connect to the various organs, glands, tissues, and blood vessels.

Dyskenesia can be quantified through range of motion analysis using a dual digital inclinometer or motion imaging studies such as an x-ray, CT, or MRI.

- ***Dysafferentation*** – in simple terms, dysafferentation refers to the inaccurate perception of the environment by the nervous system. The nervous system relies on sensory input to properly perceive its environment. For example, the fact that you know the ground under your foot is level, is because mechanoreceptors and proprioceptors in the joints of your foot sent that information to your cerebellum (part of your brain). That is called sensory or afferent information. If the ground under your foot was uneven but this information did not reach your cerebellum, you would be susceptible to accidentally spraining your ankle and falling to the ground. Afferent input is how you know if your environment is warm or cold, dry or wet, loud or quiet, uphill or downhill, light or dark, etc. Afferent input is also how you can tell if the person in front of you is a friend or foe, happy or sad, offended by you or offensive toward you. Dysafferentation is the process by which a subluxation will interfere with the inflow of information to the brain and the nervous system's perception of its surroundings. Just as dyskinesia can cause degeneration and arthritis, dysafferentation can result in poor balance and coordination, as well as inappropriate behavior such as that seen in attention deficit hyperactivity disorder. Dysafferentation is a viable explanation of how a subluxation in the atlanto-occipital junction (C0-C1 joint) of Dr. Kevin's spine was causing his seizures, and why correction of that subluxation allowed for his brain to function normally. If the brain does not receive proper neurologic input from the outside environment, it cannot function normally.

- ***Neurodystrophy*** – refers to the effect of a subluxation on tissues and organs of the body with regard to the endocrine system and the immune system. According to the neurodystrophic model of subluxation, interference with the nervous system causes stress in the body, resulting in a sympathetic response and a decline in the strength of the immune system. This is the basis of disease progression in the body. As the sympathetic nervous system is altered by a subluxation, the body's response to infectious agents is also altered.

The best way to illustrate this concept is to look at a couple of research studies:

- One study showed that spinal adjustments in the upper to mid back caused an improved immune response in the subjects. The researchers measured the amount of neutrophils in the blood. Neutrophils are the most abundant type of white blood cells and they function to rid the body of harmful bacteria, fungi, and other foreign material. The results of the study showed that only 15 minutes after the adjustment there was a significant increase in the white blood cell count as compared to blood neutrophil levels prior to the adjustment.[2]

- In a different controlled study, HIV positive patients were used as subjects to study the effect of chiropractic adjustments on the immune system. The HIV (Human Immunodeficiency Virus) attacks and destroys CD4 cells. CD4 cells, also known as T-Lymphocytes, are a type of white blood cells that play a major role in protecting your body from infection. They detect viruses and bacteria and in response signal the activation of the immune system. Patients infected with HIV gradually lose all of their CD4 cells and become completely immune compromised. In this research study, chiropractic adjustment of the upper neck resulted in a 48% increase in CD4 cells, while the control group (subjects who did not receive the chiropractic adjustments) experienced a 7.96% decrease in CD4 cells.[3]

Based on the research, the nervous system is directly involved in the control and monitoring of the immune system and therefore any interference in the function of the nervous system will directly affect the body's ability to prevent disease and recover from an illness. Remember from the last chapter that almost all healing, repair and regeneration of bodily tissues (i.e. muscles, bones, organs, glands, and blood vessels) occur while the body is in the parasympathetic state of the nervous system. Also remember that negative stress causes a sympathetic response. Therefore, according to the scientific evidence, sustained and continuous negative stress that is caused by a spinal subluxation will over time significantly reduce the body's ability to rest, repair, regenerate, and heal itself. It is of absolute vital importance to regularly monitor the spine for subluxations and get adjusted at the first detectable sign of spinal subluxation.

## Subluxations

If you decided not to read the last few paragraphs or if you would like a little simplification, here's a brief explanation without the complexities. A subluxation can begin with either a misalignment or immobility (fixation) of a bone in the spine. This will lead to degeneration of the disc and joints at that particular level. As degeneration progresses, discs will bulge, bones will form bone spurs, and the joint capsules become thicker. The bulging discs, the bone spurs, and the thickening of tissues will take up space and compromise the canal in which the spinal cord rests. The result will be painful spinal joints, eventual compression of nerves that exit the spinal column and compression of the spinal cord itself. Compression of the spinal cord or the exiting nerve roots will interfere with the brain's ability to monitor and control the organs, glands, blood vessels, muscles, and joints. In addition to pain, the end result will be gradual progressive decline in organ function and overall health, all of which could have been avoided if the health of the spine was being monitored and maintained by a chiropractor.

How does a chiropractor monitor the health of the spine and nervous system?

The most important concept to understand about chiropractic is that the focus of your chiropractic evaluation is not based on your symptoms. In fact many health conscious people including athletes and weekend warriors regularly visit chiropractors despite the fact that they have no pain or any other symptoms for that matter. Quite often I hear "Doc, I have no pain or problems; my wife just recommended that I come in and get checked for subluxations."

What does a typical first visit to a chiropractor look like?

The first thing your doctor of chiropractic will do is gather information. This may be done through online health history forms, a face to face conversation, or a combination of both.

Next, the chiropractic physical exam will be focused on looking for the common signs of subluxation. Those signs include postural abnormalities, abnormal heat patterns around the spine, swelling, pain or tenderness to touch, abnormal muscle tension or spasm, loss of range of motion, and cerebellar dysfunction as determined through abnormal balance and incoordination (clumsiness).

To objectively quantify the effects of subluxation, your doctor will most likely use computerized instrumentation. Thermography can be used to visualize the abnormal heat patterns around the spine. In a normal and healthy person, the thermal discrepancy on the sides of the spine at each segment must be minimal. For example, the temperature reading to the right of the C1 vertebra should be nearly identical to the temperature on the left side of C1. A warmer reading on one side indicates abnormal blood flow, abnormal constriction, or dilation of blood vessels, and signifies that a subluxation exists somewhere in the spine (not necessarily at C1).

Electromyography may be used to digitally measure the tension and tone of paraspinal musculature (muscles surrounding the spine). Similar to thermography, muscle tone and tension must be within normal parameters and symmetrical when comparing the right and left at each spinal level. Abnormally high muscle tone represents muscle spasm while abnormally low tone represents below normal nerve activity and neurologic weakness. Both asymmetry of muscle tone and abnormal muscle tone are indications that a subluxation exists somewhere in the spine.

Another computerized test that may be performed in the chiropractic office is digital inclinometry to accurately measure range of motion in different regions of the spine.

Limitation in motion, such as the inability to bend at the waist, is an indication of possible subluxation. Similarly, asymmetrical movement patterns, in which for example, a person cannot turn his head to the right but has no trouble turning to the left, are indicative of spinal restriction and subluxation. Certainly instrumentation is not always necessary to see limitations in range of motion. A visual assessment of how the patient bends and turns will also provide valuable information.

Finally, one of the most useful and revealing computerized tests in chiropractic is the heart rate variability analysis. The results of this test will provide information regarding the patient's ability to cope with stress. The test will compare the patient's stress adaptability to that of the ideally "healthy" person. A low score means the patient will most likely suffer ill health from stressful situations, while a high score indicates that this patient can handle a fair amount of negative stress without succumbing to illness. Furthermore, the heart rate variability test will reveal valuable information about the patient's autonomic nervous system.

Recall that the two divisions of the autonomic nervous system are the sympathetic (commonly referred to as "fight or flight") and the parasympathetic (commonly referred to as "rest and digest") nervous systems. The heart rate variability test can determine with accuracy whether a patient is predominantly in the sympathetic or parasympathetic state. Dominance in either system is undesirable. Please refer back to the previous chapter for a list of symptoms that arise from sympathetic or parasympathetic dominance.

In short, if the patient being examined is not in balance between the sympathetic and parasympathetic neurologic tone, this patient is not healthy – even if he or she has no major pathologies such as diabetes, heart disease, cancer, tumors, or autoimmune disorders. The chiropractic correction of a subluxation has been shown effective in improving heart rate variability and restoring balance in the autonomic nervous system. According to the research "The heart rate variability analysis indicates that chiropractic treatment is associated with a shift to a healthy autonomic nervous system balance."[4]

The typical first visit to the chiropractor is not complete until spinal x-rays have been taken. The x-rays allow the doctor to actually look inside the patient and see any spinal abnormality or misalignment that may be present. The x-rays will also reveal the extent of degenerative changes that may have taken place as a result of subluxation. Recall from earlier in this chapter that it may take many years of progressive spinal degeneration before such detrimental changes become visible on an x-ray. Therefore the x-rays will also allow the chiropractor to estimate the age of the subluxation.

Dan was a 60 year-old retired police officer. He sought my help because the pain in his lower back had been radiating down into his right leg, all the way to the foot. He was also experiencing extreme weakness in the right leg. He needed a cane to get around. He told me that his only grandchild was already a year old and he had never picked her up and held her because of his disability.

After reviewing his x-rays, I informed him that "based on the size of the bone spurs and the extent of disc degeneration, this problem started over 20 years ago and has been gradually progressing during the past 20 years."

Dan had a hard time accepting this. "My pain started last year, not 20 years ago," he said. "Also my medical doctor said the degeneration in my spine is a normal part of aging and since I'm getting older, I'm supposed to have arthritis in the spine."

I used the following analogy to address Dan's concern. Imagine you're driving your car and you accidentally hit a pothole. The pothole was so deep that it sounded like you damaged your car. So, you pull over and walk around your car. Everything looks normal. You kick the tires and they too seem fine. You get back in your car and start driving. There are no abnormal sounds and the car seems to be driving as before. So, you assume everything is okay. However, several thousand miles of driving later, you go in for an oil change and the mechanic says tires on one side of your car need to be replaced. You may say, "I got all four tires from the same place and at the same time, why would these two wear out and not the others?" The obvious answer would be that the pothole you hit must have thrown off your alignment. When the alignment is off, the tires wear out unevenly.

How does that apply to the spine? Well, Dan's doctor said wear and tear in the spine is a normal part of aging. The degenerative changes in Dan's spine were isolated to two of the discs in his lower back. The other discs looked perfectly healthy on x-ray. Why would two discs wear out and not the others? Aren't all of the discs the same age? Didn't Dan get all of his discs from the same place and at the same time? If degeneration and decay of spinal joints are a normal part of aging, then all of the discs and joints in Dan's spine should degenerate, not just two of them. In fact everyone who is the same age as Dan would have the same exact pattern of degeneration. But in reality, degeneration and arthritis starts at different ages in different people and it depends mainly on the person's lifestyle stresses and not their age.

So, why didn't Dan have pain for the entire 20 years? Why did he begin experiencing pain only over the past one and a half years? For the same reason that early stages of cancer have no pain and heart disease is painless until the artery gets so clogged that the heart can't function anymore. And, for the same reason that a tooth cavity initially has no pain.

Dan's story had a happy ending. It took a full year of chiropractic care, but Dan did regain full function of his right leg. Today he is spending most of his retirement playing with his granddaughter.

We know how misalignments can occur in a car, but how do they occur in the spine? Similar to hitting a pothole with your car, they can occur during childhood when we're playing in the school yard or on the monkey bars in the playground. As a child I don't recall anyone being concerned about my spine when I fell off the swing set or crashed my bike. If the bleeding stopped and I was able to move the body part, then we assumed I was fine.

Spinal subluxations can occur during the time a child learns to walk. By the time my youngest son was 15 months old, he had pretty much mastered walking but he still fell about every 15 minutes. How would you feel if you fell every 15 minutes over the next 2 hours? How about if you fell 5 times per day, every day for the next 3 months? Is it possible there would be a subluxation in your spine? Then it only makes sense to have our children checked and adjusted on a regular basis.

Spinal subluxations can also result from other trauma such as car accidents. The forces generated in a car accident are enough to tear ligaments and herniate discs. Certainly such forces will also result in misalignments of vertebrae and can cause subluxations. Once again, most people are quick to take a pill for their post-accident headache or operate on a herniated disc, but too few people pursue a chiropractic adjustment to correct their subluxations after a car accident.

Subluxations are relatively unavoidable at any age. We put pressure on our neck and spine by performing normal activities, such as sitting for a long period of time, performing repetitive movements, lifting, twisting, bending, falling, etc. It is highly improbable to avoid misaligning our vertebrae.

Spinal subluxations can even occur during birth. Being born can be very traumatic, especially to the baby's neck. Dr. Ogi Ressel discusses this "largely under-reported problem" in his book *Kids First, Health With No Interference*. "During the process of delivery, there is tremendous stress placed on the head and neck of the baby and often this stress causes vertebral subluxations of the very delicate spinal bones of the infant," states Dr. Ressel. Remember that vertebral subluxations affect the nervous system and can compromise communication between the brain and the rest of the body. It is particularly important to correct any interference at this stage of life because a newborn is rapidly developing physically, mentally, and neurologically. According to Dr. Ressel, the resulting health problems "can appear seemingly unrelated to the process of delivery and can affect your child months or years later – even as an adult!"[5]

In other words, if communication between the body and the brain is inefficient, then the development of the whole body will be affected. And, while some of the problems may be apparent immediately, others may not manifest until much later in life.

As in Dr. Kevin's amazing story at the beginning of this chapter, subluxations can cause a vast array of medical and neurological conditions. As stated earlier many infant and childhood disorders can be due to subluxations caused at the time of birth or even before that. If the mother's pelvis is misaligned, the baby can be constricted in the womb. This is called In-Utero Constraint. That means a subluxation of the baby's spine may occur even before he or she is born. Correcting these subluxations is so crucial that it should be part of the medical procedure (like the APGAR screening) for newborns. In his book, Dr. Ressel reports that "certain hospitals in Australia are now having chiropractors check infants immediately after delivery to ensure a healthy spine and nervous system free from subluxations." Maybe one day the entire obstetrics community will understand this but to date, it is the responsibility of the enlightened parents to have their infant checked for subluxations.

Subluxations in infants can be the cause for:

- Colic
- Feeding problems
- Sleeping disabilities
- Reflux
- Plagiocephaly (flat heads)
- Constipation
- Colds
- Ear Infections
- Sinus disorders

- Headaches
- Asthma
- Allergies
- Behavioral disorders
- ADD/ADHD
- SIDS (Sudden Infant Death Syndrome)
- And many, many more conditions.

The experts agree, that birth can cause trauma to the brain stem and the upper neck of the baby. Furthermore, they agree that constriction of the brain stem and the upper portion of the spinal cord, can affect the respiration and the respiratory control center of the baby. This negatively affects the baby's ability to breathe properly while asleep. This is how a subluxation resulting from a traumatic birth can cause Sudden Infant Death Syndrome. [6,7,8]

In an article entitled "Subluxation and Sudden Infant Death Syndrome," Dr. Christopher Kent has done an excellent review of the research pertaining to this subject. The data clearly states that not only can a traumatic birth cause a subluxation but that most newborns do not display any signs and symptoms of the subluxation until later. In his article, Dr. Kent cites several sources stating that a subluxation at the top of the spine has been linked to Sudden Infant Death Syndrome (SIDS). Subluxations resulting from traumatic birth can also cause "symptoms of irritability, colic, failure-to-thrive syndromes, and those syndromes associated with lowered immune responses." [9]

In another article entitled "Pediatric Chiropractic in the 21st Century," Dr. Christopher Kent discussed the findings of German medical physicians Dr. G. Gutman and Dr. H. Biederman. These doctors conducted extensive research on nerve dysfunction in newborns. They found that 80% of all newborns have a subluxation in the upper segments of their spine. They reported that common symptoms associated with spinal subluxation in newborns included "sleeping disorders, fever of unknown origin, loss of appetite, central nervous system disorders, and asymmetric motor patterns." They concluded that the subluxations were the cause of many other symptoms in newborns and had long-term repercussions throughout the baby's childhood and adult life.[10]

Dr. Kent also cites research involving infantile colic and asthma. "A prospective, uncontrolled study of 316 infants with infantile colic showed a satisfactory result in 94% of cases receiving chiropractic care." Dr. Kent further stated that the results occurred within two weeks of starting chiropractic care. Regarding asthma, Dr. Kent referenced an article entitled "Chiropractic response in the pediatric patient with asthma: a pilot study." The results of this study showed that "seven of the eight patients who completed the study were able to reduce or discontinue medication." Clearly, based on the data and the published research, correction of subluxations in the pediatric patient is of paramount importance.[11, 12]

In her research on 1,250 five-day-old babies, Dr. V. Fryman found that 95% of them had subluxations after birth. In addition these infants also suffered from muscle strain in their neck. Her research reported that the babies had immediate muscle relaxation and better sleep after being adjusted.[13]

Too often, a parent's first inclination is to seek out traditional medicine when dealing with childhood health conditions. Unfortunately, the only help they receive is in the way of medications. When an infant is seen by a chiropractor, their subluxations are adjusted manually, and with a very light touch. The results can seem miraculous, and the truth is that once the neurologic communication is restored, the body will function at optimal levels.

Let's review why an entire chapter is dedicated to chiropractic in a book about stress.

- Chapter One said *more important than stress is the body's ability to adapt to stress.*
- Chapter Two stated that *environmental stressors are what determine how your genes express themselves.*
- Chapter Three showed that *the interface between the outside environment and the DNA is the nervous system.*
- In this chapter I revealed the reality that *spinal subluxations will negatively interfere and suppress the function of the nervous system, thereby changing our genetic expression, and ultimately reducing our ability to adapt to our stress-filled environment.*
- The best way to ensure your nervous system is always optimally tuned is by routinely having your spine checked and, when necessary, adjusted by a chiropractor.

So let's put it all together. If my spine is subluxated, there is a high probability that I know nothing about it, but while I'm unaware, the subluxation is negatively affecting the inflow of information from the environment to my brain. It is also causing a sympathetic response which is weakening my immune system, interfering with my ability to rest/sleep, and decreasing my adaptability to stress. Misinformation leads to different patterns of gene expression, which leads to the potential of more disease and illness and in turn, can lead to a downward spiral in health. It is a vicious cycle that continually diminishes my ability to properly respond to stress.

You cannot prevent subluxations. And regardless of your age, or health status, you can always benefit from chiropractic care. It doesn't matter that you haven't seen a chiropractor recently (or ever), what matters is what you do today. There are a multitude of health conditions that can be rectified, prevented, or at least improved upon by beginning to take care of your spine. Getting rid of misalignments will improve function and provide you with enormous health benefits.

Therefore, the most vital and valuable action you should take with routine regularity to StressProof your life, is to get adjusted.

Sources:

1. Kent C. Models of Vertebral Subluxation: A Review. Journal of Vertebral Subluxation Research, August 1996, Vol 1, No 1, Pg. 1-7.

2. Brennan PC, Triano JJ, McGregor M, et al. Enhanced neutrophil respiratory burst as a biological marker for manipulation forces: duration of the effect and association with substance P and tumor necrosis factor. J Manipulative Physiol Ther 1992; 15(2):83.

3. Selano JL, Hightower BC, Pfleger B, et at. The effects of specific upper cervical adjustments on the DC4 counts of HIV positive patients. Chiropractic Research Journal 1994; 3(1):32.

4. Zhang J, Dean D, Nosco D: Effect of Chiropractic Care on Heart Rate Variability and Pain in a Multisite Clinical

Study. Journal of Chiropractic Education. Vol. 19, No. 1, 2005

5. Ressel, Ogi, *Kids First, Health With No Interference*, Garden City Park: Square One Publishers, 2006. Print.

6. Bonci A, Wynne C: "The interface between sudden infant death syndrome and chiropractic." *Journal of Chiropractic Research* 1989 5(3):78.

7. Stiga J: "Sudden infant death syndrome." *American Chiropractor* October 1983:28.

8. Banks B, Beck R, Columbus M, et al: "Sudden infant death syndrome: a literature review with chiropractic implications." *J Manip Physiol Ther* 1987 10(5):246.

9. http://www.subluxation.com/subluxation-and-sudden-infant-death-syndrome/

10. http://www.subluxation.com/pediatric-chiropractic-in-the-21st-century/

11. http://www.subluxation.com/subluxation-and-sudden-infant-death-syndrome/

12. http://www.subluxation.com/pediatric-chiropractic-in-the-21st-century/

13. Bladt, Dorte, D.C. "Get Ahead Kids® Feature ArticleGet Ahead Kids - Vol. 5, No. 5 - September/October 2013." Babies & Chiropractic. Get Ahead Kids, Sept.-Oct. 2013

# Chapter 5
## *The Simple Seven*

*"Simplicity is the ultimate sophistication."*

- Leonardo da Vinci

## *Seven Simple Ways to Improve Your Stress Adaptability*

In addition to getting adjusted there are some very practical ways that you can begin to improve your own stress adaptability and increase your level of wellness leading to a StressProof Life. As you read these suggestions, ask yourself, which of these can I begin doing today? I promise you that these recommendations will not require a lot of time out of your schedule to complete. So don't just read them. Underline, circle, and highlight them and create a plan that you can begin to implement today.

## <u>Light</u>

The first of the Simple Seven is light. I'm speaking about natural sunlight. In our current culture we have been taught that sunlight exposure is unhealthy. Television and internet advertisements as well as "public service announcements" are full of warnings about how sunlight may cause wrinkles and skin cancer. Such claims are simply not true. Research shows that spending time in the sun is one of the most powerful methods of fighting disease. This research shows that sunlight can help us to prevent illness such as:

- Heart disease
- Cancer
- Auto-immune disorders
- Asthma
- Digestive disorders
- And even painful conditions such as fibromyalgia.

This information is best explained in the book *Dark Deception* by Dr. Joseph Mercola.[1]

I strongly urge you to read this book. Dr. Mercola does an excellent job of comparing current research with common medical practice to reveal the myth about sun exposure. One of the startling facts he talks about is that sunlight will actually reduce your risk of cancer while most commercial sun screen lotions actually increase the risk of skin cancer.

I am not saying that sunlight cannot cause skin damage. Anyone who has had a sunburn knows that the rays of the sun are full of energy and that anything healthy can also be harmful in excessive doses. A sunburn can certainly trigger the onset of skin cancer but there is no evidence that sun tanning that does not result in a burn will have the same effect.

In his book, Dr. Mercola states that there is no evidence that sunscreens actually prevent melanoma in fact, he cites research that states populations in higher latitudes where there is less sunlight have a higher prevalence of melanoma. Meanwhile, those who spend more time in the sun tend to have a lower probability of developing melanoma. "Careful sunbathing has the potential to radically reduce many of the chronic degenerative diseases that rank among the greatest health problems faced by modern man," states Dr. Mercola.

The basis for such claims is the fact that the body produces vitamin D when the skin is exposed to sunlight. According to an article published by the Mayo Clinic on October 1, 2011, as little as 10 minutes of sun exposure per day may be enough to prevent vitamin D deficiencies. Apparently the Mayo clinic agrees with Dr. Mercola because in the article they state "Recently, research also suggests that vitamin D may provide protection from osteoporosis, hypertension (high blood pressure), cancer, and several autoimmune diseases." In case you are wondering what autoimmune diseases are, here are some examples:

- Multiple Sclerosis
- Type I Diabetes
- Rheumatoid Arthritis
- Psoriasis
- Lupus
- Inflammatory bowel diseases such as:
    - Crohn's disease
    - Ulcerative Colitis

In his book, Dr. Mercola also states that vitamin D produced as a result of exposure to sunlight may prevent the devastating effects of Alzheimer's disease.

So, why am I insisting that we get our vitamin D from the sun instead of just taking vitamin D supplements? First of all, anything accomplished naturally is far superior to its synthetic counterpart. Secondly, there are potentially dangerous side effects that can result from an overdose of vitamin D taken orally. The human body is able to self-regulate and it is highly unlikely that the body will produce toxic doses of vitamin D as a result of sun bathing.

On the other hand taking vitamin D supplements requires that you closely monitor your blood vitamin D levels through laboratory testing to ensure proper dosing. Finally, some synthetic vitamin D supplements have been proven ineffective which makes them a complete waste of money.

If that isn't enough reason to spend moderate amounts of time in the sun, consider the fact that sunlight also helps the body regulate its natural mood stabilizing hormones and neurotransmitters such as serotonin. According to WebMD, published on December 5, 2002, "A new study shows that the brain produces more of the mood-lifting chemical serotonin on sunny days than on darker days." Serotonin is the body's natural anti-depressant. In this article the researchers stated that the level of serotonin in the blood was directly related to the number of hours of sunlight in the day.

Earlier I mentioned that the suggestions I give you in this chapter will be practical, easy to implement into your daily life, and will not require much additional time out of your schedule. You may not have the time to spend 15 minutes sunbathing every day. You may live in a climate that has limited hours of sunlight. You may not have the resources to migrate south for the winter every year. So, let's talk about the practical applications of this information and how we can get more exposure to sunlight in a safe manner.

One quick way to increase healthy sunlight exposure is to not wear sunglasses. Obviously looking directly at the sun is terribly detrimental to your eyes. Also glasses will protect your eyes from flying debris when riding a motorcycle or a convertible car. So, take the necessary precautions. However, if you are walking from your car to your office, in the parking lot of a grocery store, or going out to check the mail, it's a good idea not to wear sunglasses. We absorb a high level of the sunlight we need through our eyes and unfortunately, glass and plastic both block 100% of the healthy ultraviolet (UVB) rays of the sun. Whenever possible, wear shorts and short sleeve shirts and try not to cover your face when going outside. Do not wear sunscreens unless you are going to be in the sun for an extended period of time and be sure to use natural organic sunscreens. Dr. Mercola's book *Dark Deception* is an excellent reference to use for sunscreen information.

Finally, if none of the above suggestions are practical for you, here is one last option to improve your natural vitamin D and serotonin levels. Use full spectrum lighting at home or in your office. Full spectrum light bulbs are easy to find. Typically full spectrum light bulbs come in the form of fluorescent bulbs or tubes. A search on the internet can quickly help you find a desk lamp that provides you with full spectrum lighting. Always have a full spectrum light lamp on your desk when working. If possible change all the light bulbs in your home to full spectrum light bulbs. Although, as mentioned before nothing artificial will ever fully replace the real thing, natural spectrum light lamps can be a safe alternative.

## Visualize

When dealing with psychological stress, there are few tools that are easier than visualization. In addition to the psychological dimension, this technique will have a significant impact in the physical and biochemical dimensions of stress as well. Visualization is a type of meditation. In an article entitled "*Meditation: A simple, fast way to reduce stress*" the Mayo Clinic stated "Meditation can give you a sense of calm, peace and balance that benefits both your emotional well-being and your overall health.[2]

And these benefits don't end when your meditation session ends. Meditation can help carry you more calmly through your day and can even improve certain medical conditions." The same article by the Mayo Clinic stated that some research suggests that meditation can help with common conditions such as:

- Allergies
- Anxiety disorders

- Asthma
- Binge eating
- Cancer
- Depression
- Fatigue
- Heart disease
- High blood pressure
- Pain
- Sleep problems
- Substance abuse

The important thing to remember is that meditation is not a treatment of any specific condition. Meditation is a tool that will increase and improve your ability to handle stress in the three dimensions of life.

Understandably, the term meditation can be intimidating to some and it may seem more complicated than it should be. A simple visualization exercise may take less than 60 seconds to accomplish. For example, just imagine yourself on vacation. In your mind, return to a place where you experienced some of your fondest memories, and relive those moments. Remember who was with you and what it felt like to be there. Remember the sights and scenery. Remember the sounds and the smells.

Close your eyes and really pretend that you have actually gone back to your favorite place. If it's the beach that you like, then pretend you can hear the waves crashing and sea gulls squawking. Pretend you can feel the breeze in your hair and feel the sun in your face.

You may also choose to go somewhere you've never been. You may want to climb K2 or hike the Appalachian Trail. You can go island hopping in the Caribbean or scuba diving in the South Pacific. You can play golf on the world's most exotic golf courses. You can go one-on-one with Michael Jordan or score the winning goal in the World Cup Championship game. Even the sky isn't the limit. You can go to outer space or other planets.

Set a timer for one minute and begin visualizing. Try it right now. After 60 seconds, return from your virtual vacation feeling refreshed and rested. Do this exercise at least once per day and on more stressful days you can do this every hour if you like. The only requirement is that you make it as real as possible. You must visualize every imaginable detail while on your virtual vacation. It has to feel as if you are really there. Also, during this 60 second vacation, you are not allowed to think about work, emails, bills, meetings or appointments. Just tell yourself they will be waiting for you when you're done and you'll attend to them then. The health benefits of this exercise are extraordinary and as I promised earlier, it hardly requires any time out of your schedule.

Research shows that the mind cannot tell the difference between an actual event experienced and one that is vividly imagined in detail. Therefore the outcome on a physiologic level is the same even when you only imagine the experience. Experiments performed on high level athletes prove this. Sensors were placed on various muscles throughout the bodies of Olympic figure skaters. The athletes would then visualize their routine while the sensors recorded motor nerve activity using electromyography. Motor nerves are the nerves that cause muscles to contract in sequence to produce the outcome of movement and athletic performance. According to this research, the motor nerve activity during visualization was identical to when the athlete actually performed the exercise on ice.

Another research study on this subject was conducted by Dr. Blaslotto at the University of Chicago. This time the subject of the study was basketball players shooting free throws. Initially, the free throw percentage of the basketball players were accurately measured and recorded. Then the players were randomly divided into three groups. The first group of players practiced shooting free throws for one hour a day for 30 days. The second group spent an hour a day only visualizing shooting and making free throws. The third group was considered the control group. They neither shot free throws nor visualized the process.

After 30 days of doing nothing, the third group showed no change in their free throw shooting accuracy. The first group that was allowed to practice shooting free throws for an hour a day, showed a 24% improvement in their free throw shooting. The second group of players, who only visualized making free throws, demonstrated an astonishing 23% improvement in their shooting accuracy. This was accomplished without ever physically touching a basketball.

Is there an area in your life where you could benefit from a 23% improvement in accuracy? Begin visualizing. If visualization is this powerful in athletic performance, it will certainly work wonders for you in managing stress.

Dr. Bernie Siegel is the author of several books including the famous bestseller *Love, Medicine, and Miracles*. In this book he writes about his experience as a general and pediatric surgeon as well as his vast experience working with thousands of cancer patients. Dr. Siegel was able to accomplish miraculous results in cancer patients through visualization techniques. Patients who were expected to die within a few weeks of being diagnosed with cancer were able to survive and continue a productive life for many years thanks in part to Dr. Siegel's visualization techniques.

Dr. Siegel used imagery to assess the mental state of his cancer patients. When working with children, he would ask them to draw a picture of their disease, or a picture of their doctors, nurses, or treatment methods, etc. Through these experiments, Dr. Siegel discovered that the pictures the kids drew could be used as an indicator or even a predictor of how they would respond to their treatments. For example if a child drew a "skull and bones" symbol on the radiation therapy equipment, it meant that the child had a negative view of his or her therapy and therefore probably was not handling the stress of his/her illness in an effective manner. On the other hand if the child drew angel wings on the treating doctor and nurse, you could tell that this child was hopeful about his recovery and probably would respond positively to his doctor's care. Dr. Siegel would then use the child's imagination and visualization techniques to improve their internal "picture" and their ability to handle the stress they were under.

Dr. Siegel's books are full of emotionally charged and inspiring stories of how his patients were able to overcome serious health challenges through such techniques. His books will also provide you with tools and examples of different types of visualization and meditations you can use in the convenience of your home. I highly recommend that you begin by reading Love, Medicine, and Miracles.

Our brains are capable of conducting simulations that are far more complicated than any man-made computer. Have you ever had a dream or nightmare that seemed real? People have reported waking up from a nightmare drenched in sweat or feeling tired as if they had been running. Others have reported having sore muscles after waking from a dream in which they performed physically strenuous activity. Once again this proves that the human mind is more powerful than we can imagine. There is healing power there that is not always being utilized by those who need it the most. Don't wait until life stress causes illness in your body. Use daily 60 second visualizations to increase your body's adaptability to stress so that your stress becomes a stimulus for making you stronger and healthier. And if you do encounter an illness, use visualization tools to improve your health.

One Sunday morning at church, the pastor shared the following story. Cliff was a morbidly obese man, sadly confined by his weight to his home. He had attempted to lose weight many times, tried every diet on the planet, and was still unsuccessful. You and I might have many thoughts as to why he struggled and things he might not have tried, however, I think it's safe to say, he had probably heard those ideas and many more. One day someone presented Cliff with an idea he had never considered. Although skeptical, he agreed, as it seemed like something easy enough to implement. All he had to do was listen to a series of audio programs as he drifted off to sleep every night. He was to listen to one session per night and when he had listened to all of them, he was to start over and begin again.

Cliff did as instructed. After a period of time he found that not only had his eating habits changed, so had his thoughts and desires. He actually lost over 100 pounds with relatively little effort. He was still significantly overweight but now he was able to leave his house and run errands independently. One day he was in the grocery store pushing his shopping cart, when a little boy at the end of the isle exclaimed "Mommy, look at the fat man." The embarrassed mother tried to hush and move the young boy along but could not keep him from pointing directly at Cliff. However, Cliff found himself turning side to side searching for the enormous man that the little boy was fascinated by. It took him a moment to realize that the little boy had been pointing directly at him. You would imagine that this would be hurtful but Cliff was thrilled to realize that his image of himself had changed so drastically that he no longer viewed himself as fat. He credits the audio program with reprogramming his mind and helping him change his self-image. He believes that the reason he was now able to lose weight was that he had created a new mental identity for himself in which he was thin. It was only his body that had to catch up to that image and it was doing just that.

Just like Cliff, you can use visualization to clarify your own self-image. Find out what motivates you and focus on that. Do not allow negativity, fear, doubt, and worry to enter your mind.

"Whatever the mind of man can conceive and believe, it can achieve." – W. Clement Stone

## Move

I don't mean pack your bags and move. By move I am referring to actual physical motion. Being sedentary is extremely detrimental to your health. Life is motion and motionless is equivalent to death. Incorporate motion in your daily life. Ideally, you should exercise for 30 to 45 minutes per day but earlier I promised you that anything I mention in this chapter will not require a great amount of resources such as time and money. Therefore, let's discuss ways to incorporate movement into your life. Any movement is beneficial.

# The StressProof Life

Here are some simple ideas:

- Take the stairs instead of the elevator whenever possible.

- Park at the far end of the parking lot and force yourself to walk further when you go shopping.

- If you work at a desk in an office building, drink enough water that you have to go to the restroom every couple hours. Then, choose to go to the farthest restroom, preferably on a different floor and take the stairs.

- Move as much as you can as often as you can.

If your life is already hectic then finding extra time to force-fit a 45 minute workout can actually cause more harm than good. Especially if that involves a 15 minute commute each way to the gym, time to socialize with your gym buddies, and then time to shower and get cleaned up. A 45 minute workout can actually take close to 2 hours out of your schedule.

If exercise is something you want to commit to doing daily, you must make it easy to fit into your life. Imagine if brushing your teeth would take over an hour to do each day. Would you really do it twice a day, every day? If brushing teeth was that time-consuming I think more Americans would resort to dentures. Don't visualize that one!

Perhaps that's not a very realistic example, but consider why most Americans don't eat a healthy and well balanced breakfast every day. It is because they don't have time to prepare it. That's why we tend to resort to the unhealthy choices like cereal or granola bars. It is possible that some cereals and some granola bars can be somewhat healthy (depending on your definition of healthy), but they are not healthy replacements for breakfast. Yet skipping breakfast, in my opinion is even more unhealthy.

In the same way a short 3 minute workout before your morning shower may not be the most ideal and healthy scenario but it is always better than no exercise at all. So let's discuss 3 minute options for daily exercise.

Rhythmic, repetitive exercises will not only benefit your cardiovascular system, but they will also help to synchronize your biorhythms. Everything in your body runs on cycles and has a rhythm. Negative stress in its three forms (physical, chemical, and emotional) will wreak havoc on those biologic rhythms. For example, you'll notice that the minute you become emotionally stressed, your breathing rhythm will become altered and you may even tend to hold your breath. So consider doing rhythmic repetitive exercises like with a jump rope or hula-hoop. Spend just 3 minutes in the morning jumping rope. Don't take any breaks. You can rest after your 3 minutes.

Set your stop-watch and begin. Don't stop until the 3 minutes are up. Jumping jacks are not as beneficial but if you don't have rope and you don't have a hoop, they are the next best thing. The only requirement is that the exercise must have a rhythm to it.

Another example would be doing a dance sequence over and over to a 3 minute song. Play your favorite dance song and do something repetitive for three minutes. You must have rhythm and you must stay on beat.

Other 3 minute exercise options include exercises that build strength and coordination. Suggestions would be pushups, pull-ups, lunges, and squats. Your entire workout could be just seeing how many pushups you can do in three minutes. Aim high! You can purchase an inexpensive pull-up bar that fastens to a door frame to do pull-up exercises. Use a chair to assist you if you cannot do full pull-ups on your own. The next day you can count how many squats you can do in 3 minutes and another day you can do lunges for 3 minutes. Keep track of how many you did and work to increase your repetitions with each workout.

Isometric exercises will also be of great benefit to your health. Isometrics are exercises during which the joints don't move and the muscle length does not change. There is no movement during these exercises. You simply hold a difficult position for as long as you physically can. Examples include wall squats and the abdominal plank exercise. There are several variations of each of these exercises. For example, wall squats can be made easier or more difficult by changing the angle of your knees. The more advanced person can do single leg wall squats or weighted wall squats where you hold a set of heavy dumbbells in your hands during the exercise. Your entire workout would be to hold a certain position for the full 3 minutes.

In addition to the above mentioned exercises, you can choose your favorite yoga pose and hold that for 3 minutes or get into a deep martial arts stance and hold that for 3 minutes. Be sure to choose a position or exercise that is difficult for you. It should be something that initially you can only hold for 1 minute and challenge yourself to be able to do it for the entire 3 minutes. Then make the exercise harder and shoot for 3 minutes again.

You will notice that I didn't go into much detail on the specific exercises and how to perform each one. This is because this book is not on how to exercise. This chapter is still about StressProofing your life. There are countless credible books and magazines on the subject of exercise and fitness. There are gyms that offer exercise classes and there are personal trainers that would be happy to help you learn more about the human body with respect to exercise. Even a simple search on the internet will provide you with more information than you could imagine. So, instead of getting into a long and complicated discussion on the physiology and science of exercise, I have given you a brief breakdown of what you should be concerned about when exercising.

Remember that in order for your 3 minute workout routine to be effective, it has to be challenging for you. Be sure to do one of the rhythmic repetitive exercises at a rate of every other day. In between those days, be sure to do something that challenges your strength, endurance, and coordination. Maintain variety in your routines and never do the same exercise twice in a row, even if you took a day off in between. Keep a journal of your workouts and record how you performed in each exercise. For example, write down that you did 95 pushups in three minutes today or that you only had to stop 4 times during your three minute jump rope session. Compare your performance to the previous workouts and track your progress. Your objective is to see the numbers improve with each workout.

If you are absolutely honest you will admit that most mornings you don't want to get up and exercise, even if it's only 3 minutes. In fact when it comes to choosing to stay in bed, or drinking coffee in front of the TV, or reading the newspaper, as compared to doing a 3 minute workout, the others always win. So then, it's not truly the length of time that limits us. Not many people in this world are so busy that they can't spare 3 minutes out of their 24 hour day. Let's face the fact that this is a matter of laziness. I personally have used every excuse you can think of. I have heard myself say that I'm not a morning person or that my body can't do anything unless I've had my coffee, or I really need those last three minutes of sleep. I have heard them all and I have used them all.

Countless times, I have gone to bed saying "tomorrow I'm going to jump out of bed at 5:00 AM and run downstairs and exercise." Then my alarm goes off and I say "I think I will handle my stress much better today if I sleep a bit longer." You will not feel rested and ready for stress if you sleep a bit longer because your sleep has already been interrupted. You will however, feel refreshed and accomplished if you do your workout and take a shower.

Getting out of bed must be a priority and be matched with something you greatly value. For example, I value my relationship with my 2-year-old son and his well-being is a priority to me. Therefore, if he wakes up at 4 in the morning and calls out to me for help, I will have no trouble getting out of bed to help him. If my health is a core value to me and my workouts are a priority, then getting out of bed at 4 in the morning to workout should be just as easy as getting up to check on my son. When your core values come into alignment with your priorities, stress becomes tolerable. This is a principle of success in any dimension of life.

The problem is that in the morning, logic fails and emotions prevail. Know that you are ruled by your emotions and attempting to use logic to motivate your lazy sleepy butt out of bed never works.

Here is a scenario to consider. Imagine you are sound asleep at 5 in the morning and you are suddenly woken up by the sound of your smoke detector alarm. Then you notice that it's difficult to breathe because your house is filled with black smoke. Will you roll over and go back to sleep? Will you say, "I just need 5 more minutes of sleep?" Of course not! Because you are ruled by your emotions and the emotion in this scenario is fear. That fear will move you to fly out of bed and rescue your family and it doesn't care if you only slept 3 hours that night.

What other emotions do you think would provide the motivation to start your day with action? Think of something that will get you emotionally charged. Play the Rocky theme song through your alarm clock when you wake up. Go ahead and admit it, you love Rocky! Join a "Biggest Loser" contest with your co-workers. Competition is a great emotional motivator. You can also just choose to get angry at your current state of affairs and get emotionally disgusted with laziness.

Use affirmations throughout the day to stay motivated. Create a mantra that defines who you want to be and repeat it in your head over and over. Like Mohammad Ali, keep telling yourself "I am the greatest!" I may not agree with everything Mohammad Ali said, but he was an absolute master at using affirmations to maintain an emotionally charged state which motivated him to train harder than anyone else.

So, forget about using logic to convince yourself to exercise. Get emotional about it. Stop being a slave to your body's selfish demands and instead make your body your servant. One that serves your goals, dreams and desires. You don't exist to serve laziness; you exist to live life and accomplish great things. Be strong, be courageous, stand firm, have faith, and move forward with conviction. Do this and nothing will stop you.

## Supplements

By definition, supplements are meant to be supplemental to a good diet. The first question to answer would be, are they necessary? According to an article by the Harvard School of Public Health, "A daily multivitamin is a good way to make sure you're getting all the nutrients you need to be healthy."[3]

It is a proven fact that proper nutrition can help in preventing many fatal diseases such as cancer and heart disease. It is also a proven scientific fact that proper nutrition is partially responsible for optimum health, superior athletic performance, and ideal brain function.

The Mayo Clinic states that nutritional needs should be met primarily through a diet that is balanced and includes sufficient fruits and vegetables. "For some people, however, supplements may be a useful way to get nutrients they might otherwise be lacking," writes the Mayo Clinic Staff.[4]

So Harvard School of Public Health and the Mayo Clinic, as well as most other health authorities, agree that there is benefit to nutritional supplements. The difference is that some believe you can obtain everything you need in a balanced diet while others believe that it is impossible to constantly and consistently maintain a healthy nutritious diet in America today. I tend to agree with the latter. I wouldn't say that it is "impossible" to obtain all of your necessary nutrients from food sources. It just requires a great deal of work and diligence.

One reason I recommend supplements is the depleted soils in our farmlands. In ancient times farmland had to be "rested" every few years so that it could be replenished with the proper minerals. Unfortunately this is not practiced in most farms in America. Some organic farmers do practice "crop rotating" to protect the soil from mineral depletion. However, it isn't common practice on all organic farms.

I travel abroad quite often and I've noticed that fruits and vegetables in third-world countries taste so much better than they do here in the U.S. I believe the reason for this is that they practice the more primitive farming techniques and their soils remain rich in nutrients and minerals. Of course, I have also noticed that their produce doesn't look as "perfect" and beautiful as ours here in America and in fact their produce seems to rot much faster than ours. So, it doesn't look as good but it sure tastes amazing. Just an observation!

Another reason I recommend supplements is that most produce in grocery stores have such a long transit time. Meaning they are typically shipped to your town from far away, even Hawaii, South America, or Southeast Asia. You're probably thinking, "I thought you liked fruits and vegetables from third world countries." I do like fruits and vegetables from third world countries, but only when they are fresh and harvested at the proper ripeness. Especially when I am right there to eat them. The produce that makes it over to our grocery stores was picked days or weeks prior to its peak ripeness so that it could be shipped and stocked before spoiling. When I travel to the Middle East, I see that farmers pick only the ripe fruit from the tree, box the fruit and sell it the same day in their fruit stands. Which fruit do you believe is more nutritious to our bodies? The one that was allowed to stay connected to its roots until fully ripe or the one that was plucked early and allowed to ripen while sitting on a shelf or in a box?

Finally, the third reason I take supplements daily and highly recommend them is that I am much too busy to invest the time and energy in finding and preparing foods that contain all of my daily nutrition needs. Most people today don't have the ability to devote so much time and energy to making sure that their every meal contains all of the vitamins and minerals their body requires.

Then there's the matter of skipped meals. Most people I know are too busy to sit down and eat 3 square meals a day, let alone to ensure the nutritional balance of those meals. In today's America, very few working people actually take time to prepare and eat breakfast. Lunch is usually purchased from a restaurant or deli, and dinner comes pre-made in a microwavable box. Need I say more?

As with my other recommendations in this chapter, the purpose of taking supplements is to increase your body's adaptability to stress and reduce the possibility of a negative response to stress. In other words, your supplements will help to strengthen you to be able to live and enjoy the life that you want.

So the question to answer next remains, "what type of supplements should I take?" The polls show that over half of Americans take supplements on a daily basis. That number has dramatically increased over the past several decades. However, the health of Americans has not improved over that period of time and in fact Americans are now sicker than ever before. Does that mean supplements don't work? Or does it mean that without supplements we would all be a lot worse? The answer is that most of the supplements people are taking simply don't do what they were meant to do – they don't work.

Most of the supplements on the market today are synthetic, meaning they were made from chemicals that resemble their natural counterpart. Since these vitamins and nutrients are manmade, they are not recognized as food by the body. Therefore, their bioavailability and absorbability is limited. The purpose of this segment of the book is not to get into the technicalities and the biochemistry of synthetic vitamins. My objective is to make one simple recommendation. If you want your supplements to work for you, make sure they are whole food supplements, not synthetic.

You can immediately tell the difference by reading the label. A typical synthetic multivitamin will contain ingredients such as ascorbic acid, cholecalciferol, d-alpha-tocopheryl succinate, pyridoxine HCL, you get the idea. Here is a small list of ingredients you will see on the label of a whole food multivitamin: carrots, parsley, kale, beets, cabbage, etc.

To take it even one step further, you may want to purchase your supplements from manufacturers that grow their ingredients on their own certified organic farms. Such manufacturers have the ability to further control the quality of their ingredients. One such manufacturer is Standard Process and their products are distributed through healthcare practitioners. You can find a practitioner near you by searching their web site: www.StandardProcess.com.

# Music

Music is one of the most powerful tools in managing stress. Music has a direct effect on the human physiology and psyche. You can completely change or enhance the body's chemistry through music. Music can give you energy when you are tired or bring you joy when you are depressed. It can help you calm down when you are anxious and it can get you excited when you are not feeling very motivated. The amazing part is that music can do all of this within minutes and sometimes even in seconds. So turn up the volume and whenever possible, dance.

In 1980, when I was only six years old, I was informed that one of our relatives had just been diagnosed with cancer. Back in 1980, cancer wasn't as prevalent as it is today. It was so rare that when the word cancer was spoken, everyone would take a dramatic deep breath, get wide-eyed and remain silent for a moment. In this instance the person who had been diagnosed with cancer was one of my dad's cousins and in my childhood she was one of my favorite people. She used to bring me great gifts and play with me as if she was my age. My dad told me that Aunt Simi had just been diagnosed with cancer, she had only six weeks to live, and she was on her way over to our house.

Normally when I would hear that Aunt Simi was on her way over I would get excited and start jumping around the way a child does on Christmas morning. However, this time I was scared and didn't know how I should act around her. I thought I would have to be mournful around her and not act happy. I thought I should probably try and cry in front of her to show her how sad I was and maybe that would make her feel better.

Then, Aunt Simi walked in. She was a heavy-set woman with medium to short length light brown hair. She always dressed well and wore a lot of make-up, as if she was going to a party, and this time was no different. She smiled and laughed the way she always had in the past and greeted me with a big hug and kiss, the way she always did. Then she walked over to our stereo set by the living room wall. It was one of those old large stereo systems that had a record player on top, a dual cassette player in the middle and a huge black AM/FM radio receiver underneath. The whole thing sat on top of a display case that encased our family's records and audio cassette tapes. On either side of this monster were two giant speakers that were taller than I was. Aunt Simi walked over knelt down and selected a tape out of the display case. Then she stood up, put the tape in the player, pushed play, and turned up the volume. The speakers came to life with the sounds of a song that we all knew very well. It was a famous dance song and as soon as the beautiful music started, Aunt Simi began to dance. She danced beautifully. She reached out to me and pulled me toward the middle of the living room and I started to dance with her. We danced so hard that I almost forgot the terrible news. Then she pulled my dad into the middle of the living room followed by my mom. We were all dancing and laughing until the song ended. Then as we were all still standing together in the middle of our living room, Aunt Simi said "If I only have six more weeks with you, I'm going to dance and celebrate every single day."

She did exactly that. Throughout her grueling cancer treatments she listened to music and danced every single day until she died. The music must have helped her because she stayed very positive the whole time. She kept the whole family positive the whole time. She got up and danced even when her body seemed too weak to stand.

Then all of a sudden she started to feel better and stronger. Six weeks became six months and then even longer. She did finally die of cancer, but not for another 10 years. Those must have been the best 10 years of her life because a part of each and every day was a celebration, a party.

I believe the music is what kept her alive. The music helped her body to heal. The music kept our family strong. Music can do the same for you. Do what Aunt Simi did. Turn up the volume and play your favorite song. Once a day for only a few minutes listen and let the music penetrate your soul and whenever possible get up and dance. Everyday should be a celebration and just three minutes a day can radically improve your life.

## Breathe

I am assuming that since you are reading this book, you already know how to breathe. However, many people don't know that there is a right way and wrong way to breathe. Furthermore, breathing serves more functions than just the transfusion of oxygen into the body. Breathing can serve to detoxify the body. It can relax tense muscles during stressful times and be a tool in entering meditative or hypnotic states. It can be very therapeutic in treating insomnia and most importantly breathing techniques can be used to set and regulate the body's neurologic biorhythms.

In my years of clinical practice I have met many people who simply did not know how to breathe properly. There are two parts to proper breathing. One is the actual mechanics of breathing which involves the muscles you are using and how you are using them. The second is the rhythm of your breaths and the relative ratio between inhaling and exhaling.

Let's start with the mechanical part of breathing. The main muscle used in breathing is the diaphragm. This muscle sits horizontally at the base of your rib cage. When you breathe in, the diaphragm contracts. It moves down and expands the lungs and creates a vacuum that pulls air into the lungs. When you exhale, it relaxes, moves back up to compress the lungs, and pushes the air out of the lungs.

Professional singers are masters at using their diaphragm to control the amount of air leaving their lungs thus enabling them to sustain musical notes and control sound volume properly. Becoming more conscious of the diaphragm is also essential when using breathing techniques to increase your ability to adapt to stress.

Most people naturally use the diaphragm to breathe when they are relaxed. However, during strenuous exercise we need more help to get the oxygen that the body needs and this causes us to engage auxiliary muscles. These muscles are located around the neck and around the rib cage. So, when you are relaxed and breathing properly, the only muscle that should be working is the diaphragm. When you are working hard and your body needs more oxygen like when lifting weights, riding your bike, or running, the neck and rib cage muscles contract to help the diaphragm pull more air into the lungs and then the abdominal muscles contract to forcefully push the air back out of the lungs. All of this works in unison to provide for your body's oxygen needs depending on the body's demands for air.

What does all of this have to do with stress? Well, when you are in a state of high stress, as in a state of fight-or-flight, your breathing pattern changes. Let's look at a true illustration. In 2011, I was having a business meeting in my office, sitting with a couple of bank executives. Our meeting was almost over when suddenly it seemed my desk started to move up and down in front of me and so did the chairs we were sitting in. The windows began to rattle and we heard creaking sounds from the structure of the building. The whole thing continued for a few seconds and then everything stopped. Our eyes were wide open, our hearts were racing and we were all breathing faster than before. We had just experienced an earthquake in Maryland where earthquakes are extremely rare.

Even though none of us in that meeting were performing strenuous exercise, all of us were using our auxiliary muscles to breathe. Our physiology was in a state of fight-or-flight but within another minute, when we all realized that we were safe, our breathing pattern returned to normal. The auxiliary breathing muscles relaxed and the diaphragm continued to do its job of pumping air in and out of our lungs. If we had stayed in a state of negative stress longer than just a few minutes, my neck and shoulder muscles would have developed tension and my neck and shoulders would have begun to feel stiff. If we stayed in that stated for several days, we would have developed increasing discomfort and pain in the neck, and the stiffness would have further limited the range of motion of the neck and shoulders, and eventually we could have suffered tension headaches. You can avoid all of this by paying attention to your breathing pattern.

There is one other problem that occurs during times of perceived negative stress. I mentioned earlier that the rhythm of our breathing is important to our health. First of all, everything in the body has a rhythm and the different rhythms of the body coordinate with each other through the nervous system to keep our body at optimum function and performance. Brain waves have a rhythm, the heartbeat has a rhythm, the cerebrospinal fluid that circulates around the brain and spinal cord has a specific rhythm, and even the peristalsis with which our digestive tract works has its own rhythm.

Another reason that your breathing pattern has to have a rhythm is because the lungs need time to allow for the exchange of oxygen and carbon dioxide in our blood. The blood that passes through our lungs needs time to expel the carbon dioxide and become saturated with oxygen. That means air must remain stagnant in the lungs for a period of time before it is exhaled to allow for this process to take place. The time requirement for inhaling versus exhaling needs to be a one to two ratio; meaning it should take you twice as long to exhale as it takes to inhale. For example, if it takes 2 seconds to inhale, it should take 4 seconds to exhale.

This rhythm is essential for proper oxygen saturation during rest or times of minimal physical exertion, like sitting here typing on a computer. This rhythm becomes distorted when we experience perceived negative stress. The ratio between time to inhale and time to exhale becomes one to one; meaning if it takes you 2 seconds to inhale, your time to exhale will also equal 2 seconds. During times of severe negative stress you may even find yourself holding your breath.

Most people don't have the skill or the ability to accurately control the rhythm and rate of their heart, cerebrospinal fluid circulation, blood pressure, or the rate and rhythm of the intestinal tract. However, we can all very easily control our breathing rate and rhythm and the good news is that by consciously controlling our breathing we ultimately positively affect all other biorhythms.

You only need two simple exercises to help you properly handle stress and reduce the possibility of a negative outcome from stress. First, let's work on training your body to breathe using only the diaphragm and none of the auxiliary muscles. Lie down flat on your back with your knees bent. Place one hand on your chest and the other hand on you abdomen. Breathe naturally and just observe the pattern with which your chest and your abdomen move with each breath.

Some people will notice that their chest rises every time they inhale and others will notice that their abdomen rises every time they inhale. Which one do you think is the healthy way to breathe when resting? That's exactly right, if you are breathing with your diaphragm, the abdomen is the only body part that should move when breathing. If your chest is rising on inhalation, you are using your auxiliary muscles and you may be setting yourself up for a negative stress response with ensuing health problems.

Before we discuss any stress relieving exercises, you must make sure that your body learns to properly breathe using the diaphragm. Here is your assignment. Beginning today, you must spend 60 seconds per day practicing diaphragm breathing. So, for 60 seconds lie down on the floor place one hand on your chest and the other on your abdomen. Then just breathe without allowing your chest to rise. Continue to do this for the entire 60 seconds. Once this becomes easy for you and you can do it without much concentration, then do the exercise sitting at your desk or standing in line at the post office. Within one month, this should become the new normal breathing pattern for you.

Once this happens you may move on to the more advanced exercises which I will describe next.

I mentioned that during times of stress our breathing rhythm is altered. You can battle the negative stress response by spending just a few minutes per day doing a simple breathing exercise. The exercise requires you to take just 10 deep breaths once or twice per day. During this exercise, you must stay focused on your breathing and count in your mind how long it takes you to slowly take a deep breath. You can also use the help of a stop watch but this will become impractical and unnecessary as you quickly become more skilled at this exercise.

Sit somewhere comfortable to do this exercise. I don't recommend lying down to do this because you may fall asleep. While seated comfortably, begin to inhale as you count in your mind up to a count of 5. Inhale as deep as you can and use your auxiliary muscles to fully fill your lungs with air. Then begin to exhale slowly for a count of 10 – twice as long as it took you to inhale. You can count as fast or as slow as you like as long as you keep the same pace throughout the exercise. Initially you may find that it is actually difficult to exhale slowly. This is an indication that you have been in a state of fight-or-flight for too long. If you exhale through your mouth, it becomes easier to control the rate at which air exits your lungs. Take 10 deep breathes twice per day and you will notice a major improvement in the level of stress and tension that you feel on a daily basis.

When you first begin to practice this breathing exercise, you may get lightheaded or begin to hyperventilate. If this happens, immediately stop doing the exercise for that day and begin again the next day and continue until you are able to do all 10 breathes without difficulty.

A final word of caution, do not ever do this exercise while driving. It can make you sleepy or lightheaded and those are very dangerous states to be in when driving.

The benefits of this exercise go a long way in improving the body's adaptability to stress. For example, this exercise may actually help people who suffer from acute insomnia. There may be times when you are under so much stress that you cannot shut down your mind to go to sleep at night. I have experienced this in the past when the same thoughts circle around and around in my head and I just can't fall asleep. It is a very frustrating feeling, especially when you keep looking at the clock and calculating how many hours of sleep you've lost and how important it is that you fall asleep and get a few hours of rest before your busy day tomorrow.

If you ever face such a situation, just start taking really slow and really deep breaths and follow the instructions above to maintain a one to two time ratio between your time to inhale and time to exhale. This will reset your neurologic biorhythm and you will most likely not make it to your tenth breath before you fall into a deep sleep. The important part is to make sure you breathe very deeply, as slow as you can, and maintain the rhythm of exhaling twice as long as it takes you to inhale. We will discuss proper sleep in more detail a bit later.

There is another very valuable benefit to deep breathing that I want to discuss with you. In addition to restoring the natural rhythms of the body and helping you fall asleep at night, this breathing exercise will serve to cleanse and detoxify your body. It does this by improving lymph flow through the lymphatic system. The lymphatic vessels of the body are commonly referred to as the body's sewer system. The following is an overly simplified illustration of a very complex system. Similar to the sewer system that keeps our city streets clean by removing rain water and waste, the lymph channels keep the blood clean by removing metabolic waste, transporting white blood cells, and excreting cancer cells.

So, you can imagine that the flow of lymph is extremely important to our health and wellbeing. The critical part in all of this is that the lymphatic vessels are not connected to a pump that would keep the lymph flowing through the body. There are only three ways by which the lymph system circulates and cleans the body. One is by physical exercise. Muscle contraction creates the pumping action that pushes the lymph through the vessels. The second method of lymph transport through the body is by massage. In addition to helping reduce muscle stress, massage can significantly boost the immune system by promoting lymph drainage. The third and final way of promoting lymph drainage is by taking deep breaths. Deep inspiration creates the vacuum and subsequent pressure required to pump the lymph through the channels. The more lymph we pump through our system the more toxins we will remove from the body and the healthier we will be.

In fact some researchers have gone as far to say that the only reason exercise is beneficial to our bodies it that it causes us to pump the lymph channels through muscle contraction and heavy breathing. Furthermore, researchers have discovered that one of the reasons dieting does not produce the weight loss results that we expect and hope for is that the body is unable to rid itself of toxins. As a protective mechanism, the body will store toxins in adipose (fat) tissue. If the body does not hide the toxins in fat cells, the toxins can circulate throughout the body and make us ill. Therefore, the more toxins in the body, the more reluctant the body will be to shed the fat. The result is the frustration that people experience when dieting does not produce the desired effect of weight loss. I have seen many of my patients begin to lose weight simply by breathing properly and doing this breathing exercise twice daily. A body that has fewer toxins is much more capable of handling and adapting to stress.

While we are on the subject of weight loss, see if you can answer this question. Where does fat go when it is lost? Have you ever wondered about that? It doesn't just disappear, so it has to go somewhere. Theory number one, is that it becomes energy and gets used by the body. Another theory states that it gets excreted from the body through urine and feces. Some people believe that fat is actually converted to muscle when we exercise.

As you may have guessed, all of these theories are incorrect. The chemical makeup of all organic (meaning living) material is based on the element carbon. Body fat is no different. The chemical formula of a molecule of body fat (triglyceride) is $C_{55}H_{104}O_6$. That means there are 55 carbon atoms in every molecule of fat. Since carbon is much larger than hydrogen, fat is composed of mostly carbon. When we breathe in, we take oxygen from the air. What comes out when we exhale? That's right, carbon dioxide. Oxygen goes in and carbon dioxide comes out. The most efficient way to lose fat is to exhale it.[5]

This is yet another reason for you to do the suggested breathing exercise. It regulates your biorhythms, detoxifies your body, and gets rid of fat. Who could ask for anything more?

## Sleep

Why do so many of you deprive yourselves of this one? For the same reason that you skip breakfast and miss your workouts. Everyone is too busy to sleep. You know exactly what sleep deprivation feels like and I am sure you don't like it. Sleep is when the body repairs itself. A tremendous amount of metabolic and physiologic work takes place when you sleep. I read on a blog post that physical repair takes place from 10pm to 2am and psychological repair takes place from 2am to 6am, and that is why everyone must sleep from 10pm to 6am without interruption. This author went on to say that the reason so many wackos roam the streets at night and so much crime takes place after midnight is because the people who don't sleep between 2am and 6am never undergo psychological repair. There may be some truth to that, but I don't believe that a few sleepless nights will turn you into a criminal.

I agree with the concept of going to bed at the same time every night and waking up at the same time every day. Experts claim that the body needs between 7 and 9 hours of uninterrupted sleep per night. This range was determined by measuring the levels of different hormones in the body as they respond to sleep. This can quickly become very complicated, especially when you take into account the different levels of sleep such as light non-REM (rapid eye movement), deep slow wave sleep, and REM sleep, and how each results in a different hormonal response.

Here is what you need to know; the deeper your sleep and the more time you spend in deep slow wave REM sleep, the healthier your body will be. If you don't get enough deep sleep, your cortisol levels will increase and your growth hormone levels will decline. Increased cortisol levels over time will lead to metabolic problems such as increased body fat, osteoporosis, and insulin resistance. Insulin resistance is the precursor to Type 2 Diabetes. Increased cortisol levels are also linked to mental problems such as memory loss which becomes more severe with age indicating that our amount of quality sleep seems to decline with age. Declining levels of growth hormone are linked to reduced muscle mass, decreased strength, increased body fat, suppressed immunity to infectious diseases, and overall decline in health. In summary, inadequate sleep is one of the biggest contributors of aging.[6,7]

Life has a rhythm. Biologists refer to this as the circadian rhythm. It is a 24 hour internal clock that runs automatically and can adjust and adapt to the environment based on daylight. The more rhythmic your daily routine of sleep, the healthier and more adaptable to stress your body will become.

The natural hormone melatonin is responsible for regulating your circadian clock. Melatonin is released during sleep and in the absence of light. Daylight prevents the production of melatonin. This is especially significant for people who work at night and sleep during the day. Since light blocks the production of melatonin, those of you who do shift work and sleep at odd times must absolutely make certain that you sleep in pitch black darkness. Also those of you who sleep with a night light should consider turning it off when you sleep. In fact, you should cover up the alarm clock and block the light that it emits as well.

A deficiency in melatonin will cause sleep disorders which creates a vicious cycle leading to lower melatonin levels which leads to worse sleep which further lowers melatonin. You get the point. Research shows that declining levels of melatonin increase the risk of developing degenerative diseases of the brain such as Parkinson's disease and Alzheimer's disease. It may appear that supplementation with melatonin would be a good idea, but I must caution you, as I did earlier in this chapter when discussing Vitamin D. You must consult with your healthcare professional before taking oral melatonin because it may adversely react with other conditions or medications.

The best type of Vitamin D is the type your body produces when your skin is exposed to natural sunlight. Similarly, the best type of melatonin is the type your body produces when asleep in darkness.

Several years ago, a patient of mine told me that his wife, Sally had been admitted to the hospital following attempted suicide. Sally was also a long term patient of mine and their entire family visited my office routinely for wellness checkups. They had a very stable and loving marriage with two small children in private school. From her husband's perspective their life was perfect and he could not figure out why his wife of over 12 years would have tried to kill herself.

His wife was a detective with the police department in a neighboring city. She was a decorated officer and her career had been full of commendations, awards, and promotions. Now she had been diagnosed with severe clinical depression. So, I went to the hospital to visit her.

At first she was too emotional and too embarrassed to discuss her condition with me, but as we began to discuss her lifestyle it quickly became apparent why she was clinically depressed. It turns out that she worked the night shift during weeknights. She would get home as the kids were getting up to go to school. After helping the kids get ready and dropping them off at school, she would go home and sleep until it was time to pick them up from school. She would then stay awake the rest of the day doing house chores and spending time with her children until they went to bed and she would then go back to work as a police officer.

In their master bedroom, directly over their bed was a large skylight. When building their home, they had placed it there because they wanted to be able to gaze at the stars at night. However, when she slept, from morning to the early afternoon, the sun shone brightly through that window directly on her face. Now imagine the stress of dealing with criminals on a nightly basis and risking your life for the sake of protecting the public. Then add to that stress, the deficiency of melatonin because of exposure to light during sleep. Further add the increased cortisol production of not enough deep sleep and the decline in growth hormone for the same reasons. This is the perfect storm and an explosive recipe for disaster.

She said that recently she felt like she was getting sick more often. She had noticed that she was gaining weight even though she wasn't eating more. She had also begun to experience forgetfulness, mood swings, and extreme irritability. These are classic signs of sleep deprivation. It is no wonder that she was so depressed. I quickly made several recommendations but the most effective of my recommendations was for her to begin sleeping in a different room during the day.

She started to sleep in the guest room and was able to seal the windows with heavy curtains so that no light could enter the room when she was sleeping. Within 30 days, her serotonin and melatonin levels returned to normal and she was herself again.

Today, Sally and her husband are still happily married, raising their children in a loving and stable environment, and our Ms. Detective is fully equipped to handle the stress of her job without detriment to her health. She is living the StressProof life.

The moral of the story is that sleep plays a crucial role in your ability to adapt to stress. So here are a few recommendations for you. Do your very best to get 8 hours of sleep at night and if you have to sleep during the day, make sure that you sleep in pitch black darkness. Stay consistent with your schedule of when you go to sleep and when you wake each day. Do not ingest any caffeine within 6 hours prior to going to sleep.

These are easy and simple recommendations but their impact on your health will be monumental. Soon your friends and relatives will be asking you how it is that you are able to stay so young.

## Summary: The Simple Seven

1. **Light** – Moderate daily exposure to sunlight is beneficial to your health. It results in production of vitamin D by the body which is necessary to prevent many chronic degenerative diseases as well as many auto-immune disorders. Sun exposure also stabilizes the body's serotonin levels. Serotonin is a hormone and a neurotransmitter that serves to balance and enhance your mood. It is the body's natural anti-depressant.

2. **Visualize** – The human body cannot tell the difference between an actual experience and one that is imagined in vivid detail. Go on a 60 second

virtual vacation every day. Imagine yourself in the most exotic and enjoyable places doing activities that invigorate you. When you return from your imaginary vacation, your body will act as if you just returned from a real vacation. Also visualization has been proven to improve athletic performance.

3. **Move** – My dad, Javad Rashidian, used to say with a big mischievous smile, "Any body part you don't use, you will lose." So, move every joint in your body every day. Walk every day and exercise for at least 3 minutes every morning before you do anything else. It is a good idea to do an exercise that is rhythmic and symmetrical in order to support the body's natural rhythms. The internet is packed full of helpful videos and exercise routines. Pick a few that suit your needs and abilities and cycle through them, doing a different one every day.

4. **Supplements** – it is quite difficult and impractical to obtain all of the body's nutritional needs from your diet. Therefore supplementation is a good solution. Be sure to take a multivitamin, multi-mineral, fish oil, and probiotics. The multivitamin and multi-mineral must come from natural sources such as fruits and vegetables. Therefore the supplements you purchase should say *whole food* on the bottle and the list of ingredients should be things you know and recognize, like carrots, beets, kale, and sea kelp.

5. **Music** – Consider this a multivitamin for your soul. I believe music is one of the most powerful triggers of psychological and physiological responses. It can relax you or make you tense. It can motivate you or send you into depression. I can't think of too

many things in life that can affect your physiology and hormonal make-up as quickly as music. Once per day you should listen to your favorite song and whenever possible you should dance to it.

6. **Breathe** – Take a giant deep breath right now. When your lungs are full of air, just hold your breath for a few seconds and then as slowly as possible, exhale through your mouth. How do you feel? Now count to 5 as you breathe in, then pause for a few seconds and begin to exhale slowly as you count to 10. Exhaling should always take twice as long as it takes you to inhale. Do ten deep breaths in this manner in the mornings and ten more in the evenings. It will help to regulate your biorhythms, detoxify your body through proper lymph drainage, and even cause you to lose a few pounds of excess body fat.

7. **Sleep** – Do this only if you ever feel tired! Sleep is when your body does most of its repair, regeneration, and growth. Take sleep very seriously. There is a huge amount of science behind the intricacies of the sleep process but it wouldn't be part of the simple seven if it wasn't simple. It all boils down to the following few practical recommendations. Do your best to go to bed and wake up at the same time every day. Get between 7 to 9 hours of sleep every night. Sleep in pitch black darkness whenever possible, and do not ingest any caffeine within 6 hours of going to sleep. Here's one final suggestion. Take a 10 minute nap at 4 pm every day to increase your growth hormone levels. It's called a "beauty nap."

Congratulations to you for reading this far. I expect that you are making plans to incorporate all that you have learned. It all boils down to the following three keys:

A. Trust your innate intelligence
B. Get adjusted regularly
C. Do the simple seven

## Sources:

1. http://www.amazon.com/Dark-Deception-Discover-Benefits-Sunlight/dp/0785221824/ref=sr_1_fkmr0_1?ie=UTF8&qid=1434320407&sr=8-1-fkmr0&keywords=dark+deception+by+joe+mercola

2. Mayo Clinic Staff. "Meditation: A Simple, Fast Way to Reduce Stress." *Mayo Clinic*. Mayo Foundation for Medical Education and Research, 05 May 2014. Web.

3. "Vitamins." *The Nutrition Source*. Harvard School of Public Health, 2014. Web.

4. Staff, Mayo Clinic. "Nutrition and Healthy Eating." *Mayo Clinic*. Mayo Foundation for Medical Education and Research, 19 Jan. 2013. Web

5. Meerman, R., Brown A. J. (2014). When somebody loses weight, where does the fat go? *BMJ, 349* doi: http://dx.doi.org/10.1136/bmj.g7257 (Published 16 December 2014).

6. Van Cauter E, Leproult R, Plat L. Age-Related Changes in Slow Wave Sleep and REM Sleep and Relationship With Growth Hormone and Cortisol Levels in Healthy Men. *JAMA*.2000;284(7):861-868. doi:10.1001/jama.284.7.861.

7. The Journal of the American Medical Association, August 16, 2000; 284:861-868, 880-881

# Chapter 6
# *Health is Not a Destination*

*I can tell you with great certainty that the number one reason people fail to realize their dreams is that their bodies are not equipped to handle the stress that they will surely face on the road to greatness.*

We all live on a continuum between illness and health and as I mentioned earlier, every choice we make moves us in only one of two directions. We are never standing still on that continuum. We are either moving toward illness or toward wellness. So be brutally honest with yourself right now. In which direction are you moving? If the answer is that your daily habits, thoughts, and actions are moving you toward illness and away from wellness, then let this be your wake up call. Let this be the moment you make a change.

Consider the following:

Dr. Russ Reiss is a well-known cardio thoracic surgeon. In a television interview, Dr. Reiss discussed how he could usually predict which heart attack patient would recover, how quickly they would recover, and who was in danger of not surviving. He said his predictions were not dependent upon how skilled the surgeon was or how well the surgery went. He said, the outcome was mostly dependent on the patient's lifestyle up to the moment of having a heart attack. "If you live long enough, you will eventually be faced with a serious health challenge," said Dr. Reiss. That health challenge can be an illness, disease, or a serious injury. Dr. Reiss continued, "How you come out of that challenge is entirely dependent on how you've been living your life up to that moment." His point is that even those who live healthy lives will likely get sick but their chances of full recovery will be much higher if they have been living the wellness lifestyle.

In other words, according to Dr. Reiss, your lifestyle directly impacts your body's ability to overcome illness, injury, and even surgery. His message should be empowering because, although you do not have the ability to fully control when a health challenge will come your way, you do have the power to influence its outcome by StressProofing your life today.

Heath is an ever current condition of our mind and body. It can be something we are improving upon on a daily basis, but it is nevertheless something we are bound to and therefore must pay attention to. Regardless of what our circumstances have been up to now, the moment of change and improvement starts with every new day. As I said, the mere fact of not having symptoms of illness doesn't confirm that our body is healthy. Therefore our goal must be to learn all the components that get and keep us strong and incorporate these tools into our daily course of action. When we learn how to adapt to stress in a healthy manner we are fortifying our physical body, our chemical make-up, and our mental attitude.

## *Two Chiropractors Who Got Cancer*

Two chiropractors, who I know and respect, were both diagnosed with cancer a few years ago. One developed breast cancer and the other colon cancer. They were both devastated by the news of their diagnosis. It made them question everything they had done and everything they stood for. You see, both doctors were extremely fit and healthy. They exercised and ate right. They managed their lives in balance between work and home. They regularly gave lectures on how to prevent diseases such as cancer and they followed their own advice. How could they have gotten cancer?

Well, exactly one year later, both of them were cancer-free. In fact, I sat among the audience when one of them was discussing her journey and when she spoke about her battle with breast cancer, she sounded like she was speaking about a simple cold or a sore throat. Imagine facing an evil giant like cancer, slaying it, and coming out on the other side talking about it as if it was nothing. That's what the healthy lifestyle is all about.

The lesson they learned is that doing all that they did for wellness did not make them invincible, but it did give them the fighting edge they needed to be victorious. My chiropractor friends didn't know it but they were in fact preparing for the fight of their lives by living the StressProof lifestyle. Sometimes we think the only reason we do the right things is to prevent such diseases but the main reason to StressProof your life is to become stronger so that you can overcome such obstacles.

## Muhammad Ali – Are you Prepared?

Mohammad Ali once said, "The fight is won or lost far away from witnesses – behind the lines, in the gym, and out there on the road, long before I dance under the lights." Sooner or later, we will all be forced to step into the ring and our opponent may be bigger than us. We may be facing heart disease, or cancer. We may be facing stroke or multiple sclerosis. If we have been preparing and if we have been training, we have a chance at winning. Are you training? Are you prepared? If you haven't been doing this up to now, this book will hopefully help you get started.

## State Trooper Eating Chips and Soda

A few years ago, I was about to give a lecture to a group of police officers on health and stress. Outside of the building, two men were standing near the entrance. One of them was eating a bag of potato chips and drinking a can of soda. Neither of them knew that I was their next presenter. I overheard one tell the other "I can't believe we have to sit through another health class. They're probably just going to tell me to stop eating this junk, but I would rather enjoy my life and if that means I will die a few years sooner, so be it." Many people feel that way. They would rather trade in a few years of life for some short-term pleasure. That wouldn't be so bad if that's all their poor habits did. But in reality, the very thing they are trying to protect, their quality of life, is the first thing that will be taken away from them. The purpose of living a StressProof life isn't to merely prolong life. The purpose is to increase how well you live while you are alive.

### *Marlene Warren's Story* (Author of *Laugh Yourself Happy in Thirty Days*)

I started smoking late in life. I was almost nineteen at the time.  All my college buddies had years of nicotine experience behind them and I delighted in the idea that I was going to catch up. My friends tried to discourage me by saying, "Smoking was a dirty habit and I was lucky not to need a cigarette to feel cool." Cool? I had never felt cool! And anyway, I insisted that I would only smoke one cigarette a day. Two days after my nicotine initiation I was puffing away to the tune of three packs a day and that continued for thirty-five years. I loved, loved, loved smoking. When I was stressed I smoked. When I was happy I smoked. When I was sad I smoked. And you can guess what I did when I was angry.

Mornings, before becoming fully awake, I would grab a cigarette and enjoy the virgin inhale that announced the beginning of my day. As a high school teacher, when the bell rang to end the teaching period, I would push my way through the congregated students to be the first person out of the classroom to get to the teachers' lounge for my nicotine fix.

I had no intention of giving up my dastardly dirty, but delightful habit. That is until I had a medical checkup at the age of 52 with a cardiologist who checked me out and stated, 'I won't tell you to stop smoking, but I will tell you that if you keep smoking, when you're 60 years old you will wind up breathing like an eighty year old; and not a healthy eighty year old." I wasn't concerned with dying because of my smoking, but I was sure concerned with living with a substantial lack of quality of life. My moment of truth came when I realized that if I had trouble breathing and walking, I would have to choose between smoking and shopping! Shopping won and I gave up smoking.

Once again, as Marlene's story demonstrates, life is not about how long you live, it's about how superbly you live while you're alive.

## The 100 Year Lifestyle

Dr. Eric Plasker puts this issue in great perspective. He is the best-selling author of The 100 Year Lifestyle. He states that typically when asked "do you want to live to be a hundred?" most people's answer is "No!" People don't want to live to be a hundred years old because it is believed that most people who are that old are not healthy. They need help getting out of bed and going to the bathroom, and their quality of life isn't what most people want. So, why would anyone want to live to be 100 years old? Dr. Plasker states that currently the fastest growing age group is the 100-year-olds. In fact there are currently 4.2 million people in the world who are at least a hundred years old. The startling fact is that when they were born, over a hundred years ago, life expectancy was only 50. That means that they have outlived their life-expectancy by over 50 years. What was your life-expectancy when you were born? 70? 75? What if you outlive your life expectancy by 50 years? We may not have the desire to live to be 100 years old, but the truth is that we don't have a choice. The only choice we get is how healthy we are when we get there.

On November 5th, 2005, ABC's Good Morning America did a study on a man who was about to turn 100. His name is Dr. Frank Shearer. "Shearer, a retired physician in Washington state, might be the world's oldest water-skier," the reporter continued, "He also rides horses and can be seen atop a steed on the cover of this month's National Geographic magazine, which features him in an article about longevity."

"I think it has to do with the fact that I have been so active," Shearer said. "I've been active all my life, from one sport to the other sport – snow-skiing in the wintertime, water-skiing in the summertime, hunting, fishing, and especially in recent years, I've been doing some weightlifting regularly."

Like I said, you don't get to decide how long you live. You can only decide how well you live while you're alive. Do you want to be the 100-year-old who can no longer walk, or would you rather be skiing, hunting, fishing, and lifting weights when you're a hundred?

Let's discuss what it means to live well. It is similar to the definition of health. Being healthy doesn't just mean being free of pain. It means that your body is functioning optimally in all dimensions of life. Similarly living well doesn't mean avoiding junk food, drugs, and alcohol. Living well is about doing amazing things in your life. It's about experiencing life to the fullest. It's about serving your family, being a blessing to others, and leaving the world a bit better than when you found it. There's no end to it. Health is not a destination and neither is wellness.

How much do you want to accomplish in your life? How many dreams do you want to chase? How many goals do you want to reach? How many people do you want to positively influence? How successful do you want to be in your career? How strong do you want to be? How much endurance and agility do you want to have? All of those things are dependent on only one thing. They are all determined by how much stress you can handle. Recall from chapter one that I said your goal should never be to reduce stress. Your focus should be on increasing your adaptability to stress in order to decrease the probability of a negative outcome as a result of stress. In other words: *stop trying to eliminate stress and start getting stronger so you can handle more stress.*

Attempting to reduce stress is like chasing the wind. You will never catch it. The only way to reduce stress is by playing small and setting the bar low. You can easily reduce your stress by getting rid of everything that is meaningful to you. Imagine if I said having children is stressful so I'm going to give up my sons. Absolutely ridiculous! I love my boys and I would die for them. Believing that reducing stress will make you healthy is the same as believing you will get stronger in the gym by lifting less weight. You only get stronger if you challenge yourself by attempting to lift more weight.

So don't waste your efforts on reducing stress. Instead StressProof yourself. StressProof yourself by trusting your innate intelligence, getting adjusted regularly, and incorporating the *simple seven* in your daily life. StressProof yourself so that you can take the hits and still keep moving forward. StressProof yourself so you can carry that burden and not have it knock you down. StressProof yourself so you can take on the challenges that you want and succeed every single time.

You see, your level of health is entirely dependent on how much stress you can handle. If your stress adaptability is low, a little bit of stress will make you sick. If it is high, then you can handle tons of stress and you won't get sick. This is what the StressProof life will do for you. It will strengthen you so that you can take on the stress. It will enable you to take on the stress of caring for your family, the stress of succeeding in a long and fruitful career, the stress of building a legacy, realizing your dreams, and contributing to society. I have been studying the human body for the past 20 years, and I can tell you with great certainty that the number one reason people fail to realize their dreams is that their bodies are not equipped to handle the stress that they will surely face on the road to greatness.

Just as the strength of your health is dependent on how much stress you can handle, your level of success depends entirely on how much stress you can handle. Marshall Sylver, the Millionaire Maker and master hypnotist, once said, "The amount of success you achieve in life is directly proportionate to the amount of stress you are willing to embrace." Not only must you be willing to embrace more stress but your body needs to be equipped to handle the extra stress.

The size of your family and circle of friends depend entirely on how much stress you can handle. The length of your career and how far you go in that career depend on how much stress you can handle. The size of your business depends entirely on how much stress you can handle. Your income depends on how much stress you can handle. How wealthy you become and how happy you are depend entirely on how much stress you are equipped to handle. Everything that is worth having, doing, and becoming is completely dependent on your ability to handle the stress that accompanies it.

So when stress comes your way, become the kind of person who invites it. Accept stress as an ally and use it to make you stronger when fighting life's many battles. Embrace the stress, because it is a high-octane fuel that can empower you to grow in health and excel in life. Becoming StressProof is the only way you can be, do, and have all that you desire. This truly is the secret to health, wealth, and happiness.

# Chapter 7
## *Above All Else*

*"There are only two ways to live your life.
One is as though nothing is a miracle.
The other is as though everything is a miracle."*

- Albert Einstein

# The StressProof Life

On November 25th, 1995, my life drastically changed. That was the day I received a phone call from God. Sound crazy? Don't worry; this has everything to do with StressProofing your life. Let me explain.

My relationship with God began when I was only 4 or 5 years old. My mother and I used to kneel by my bed and pray. This was our routine every night before going to bed. I remember thinking that she's crazy because she spoke to someone who was invisible and I never heard Him talk back but we kept on talking to him.

"God is everywhere," my mom and dad would tell me.

"Well, can he still see me if I hide under ten blankets? If he's everywhere can we accidentally run him over with our car or shut the door on his hand by accident? How can He be here and somewhere else at the same time?"

They didn't have very good answers to those questions, but they prayed with me so much that over time I just started to believe that there was a God and that He created us. So I began to pray to Him by myself, even when it wasn't bedtime and even when no one else was praying with me.

One summer morning, I woke up to find out that it was raining. Dad had told me that if it rains we won't be going to the beach that day. I was extremely disappointed.

The large green couch in our living room backed up to a large beautiful window that faced our front yard which was actually an orchard of orange trees. As I stared out at the rain falling on the green leaves of the trees, I thought about God. I wondered if he had the power to change the weather.

"God, if you are real and you truly exist, then please make it stop raining."

Over the next five minutes, as I continued to look out the window, the rain slowly stopped, the clouds faded away and the sun came out, shining bright and beautiful. I couldn't believe it. "Thank you God." Dad and I had a great day at the beach.

A week later, I tested God again. Back then, soccer, known as football in Iran, was my favorite sport. The kids on our street and I played soccer every evening during the summer. That specific evening, we were going to go head-to-head with kids from the next street over. This game was huge because to us it was the World Cup final. The winning team would rule the neighborhood and own the bragging rights. Our team needed me. I wish it was because I was a great soccer player. In reality, it was because I had a big belly and I took up a lot of space, which made me the ideal person to play goalie.

So excited about the game, I could hardly sit still. I was really looking forward to the game, but there was one minor problem. Piano lessons! I had piano lessons three nights per week and unfortunately that night was one of them. I prayed, "God, if you are real and you truly exist, please cancel my piano lesson so that I can play in the big game tonight."

At 5 pm, the kids from the next street rolled onto our street. It looked like a showdown in the old Wild Wild West. The clash of titans was about to begin. It would be a battle of epic proportions. We started playing. I dreaded the thought of being pulled away from the game. I knew at any minute, my mother would peak her head out our front gate and wave me in for my piano lesson, but that night she never did. We finished the game and when the street lights came on, the neighborhood kids went home.

I don't remember who won the soccer game that day. What I do remember is wondering why mom hadn't called me in for my piano lesson. "What if something bad happened to Mr. Saeed?" He was my piano teacher, and I was worried that perhaps because of my prayer he had been hurt or become ill and I was feeling really guilty about it. Thankfully that wasn't the case. Apparently he had called and asked to cancel because of something unrelated to his health.

"Thank you God!" However, this time, I was terrified of the thought that my selfish desire to stay outside and play soccer may have led to someone being hurt. After that incident, I decided it was time to stop testing God. In fact I made a promise to God, that I would never again pray such selfish prayers. Ten years later, I broke that promise.

Growing up, I had two dreams. The first dream was that I wanted to become the best doctor in the world and save lives. As you may recall from the prologue, I decided to become a doctor after seeing the pregnant woman pass away in her husband's arms in the village. The second dream was to marry the most beautiful woman on the planet. As a little kid, I remember my mother and her friends looking at fashion magazines and talking about how beautiful some of the models looked. So I decided that I would one day find and marry the most beautiful girl, the girl of my dreams.

As a senior in high school, that second dream seemed like a near impossibility. I was not one of the popular kids, I was not an athlete, and I wasn't even on the chess team or in the math club. I was invisible to everyone except my four buddies. To make matters worse, I still had my big belly. During my soccer days, the belly assisted me in blocking goals, but now it only served to lower my self-esteem and destroy my confidence. To make matters worse, we didn't have much money and although I always had nice clothes, they weren't considered very fashionable by the popular kids.

Well, being invisible is not very helpful when you want Jennifer Santiago to go out with you. I had been secretly in love with her since the ninth grade but never had the nerve to ask her out. This was our senior year and I was running out of time. The homecoming dance was right around the corner and I had to act fast. There was only one minor problem. I had no idea how to talk to a girl. I had never been on a date before. I hadn't even asked anyone out on a date before.

I was going to need some serious help. "God, if you are real and you truly exist, please make sure Jennifer Santiago says yes when I ask her out to the homecoming dance." I remembered my promise that I would never selfishly test God again, but I thought this was too important to leave to chance. I swore it would be the absolute last time I did it.

I sat next to her in third period for computer science class. So, when the bell rang, I followed her out into the hallway and tapped her on the shoulder. I couldn't believe it; she actually turned around and looked at me. Perhaps I was not as invisible as I thought. This was a very good sign. The time had come to speak the words that I had spent hours writing, rewriting and rehearsing over and over. This was my moment. I froze. She kept looking at me. I thought about God and how he stopped the rain and canceled my piano lesson. Surely, He would make Jennifer Santiago go out with me. So, I nervously spoke up. "Do you want to go to homecoming with me?" Surprisingly, she didn't say no. Instead, she slowly turned around and began to walk away while I stood there. It felt like every eye in that hallway was on me. For once I wasn't invisible but really wished that I was. I thought, "My life is over and my dream will never come true. There is no reason to keep living."

I became depressed and started having thoughts of suicide. I didn't look forward to anything anymore. I was embarrassed to sit next to Jennifer Santiago in third period computer class. Worst of all, I felt like God had ignored me, or worse, He had decided not to answer my prayer. I felt completely alone. This went on for a few weeks and each day that went by, my suicidal thoughts grew stronger.

My mother had a daycare center in our home at that time. She and her assistant took care of between 6 and 8 little ones while their parents worked. My mom was phenomenal at being a part-time mom to those kids. She really cared about each one of them like they were her own. She ran that business for 22 years.

One evening, while still in my emotionally dark place, I overheard my mother speaking to one of the parents who was picking up her son after work. My mom was telling her, "Your son has learned to throw a lot of tantrums lately and the worst thing we can do is give him what he wants when he throws a tantrum." She went on to explain, "By giving him what he wants, you will reinforce that behavior and he will keep throwing tantrums to get what he wants for the rest of his life." At that moment, I had the image of a grown man sitting on the floor in the middle of a shopping mall kicking and screaming to get what he wanted. Then, it hit me like a ton of bricks. I was just like that kid throwing a tantrum. If God had given me what I asked for, I would never stop acting this way. The best thing for me was for God to ignore my selfish request.

I went to our living room and sat on the couch in front of the TV. My mother was nearby in the kitchen preparing dinner. As I sat on the couch contemplating this new revelation, I felt the need to start praying to God. So I did. I prayed with a humble heart, asking for forgiveness. I acknowledged to God that I had been throwing a tantrum and that I won't do that again. After a few minutes of praying, I asked God to give me a sign to show me that he does forgive me and that I was on the right track.

At the very moment that I asked for a sign, I looked over into the dining area of our house which was technically an extension of the kitchen, and saw the large designer mirror that hung on the wall, fall to the floor and break. That was my sign and it had come immediately after I asked for a sign. That mirror had securely hung on that wall for over 5 years. Now it was on the floor with a large crack through one corner of it. I ran over to get a closer look. Beating me to the scene, my mom was already there looking at the broken mirror.

"They say when a mirror breaks it means seven years of bad luck," she said.

"I don't think that's true in our case," I said as I ran upstairs to my room to be alone.

I was ecstatic. I had just been given a sign from God which meant he's looking out for me. I went from being depressed and fed up with life, to being enthused about the rest of my life. All the darkness and negative emotion I had been carrying with me had been lifted. I put aside my goal of meeting a girl and decided to focus on my other goal of becoming a world-famous doctor and saving lives. Classes and books became my priority and I didn't consider asking anyone out on a date again. I went to the senior prom with my group of four friends, among whom I was the only one without a date. I didn't mind. I was hopeful that when the time was right, I would meet the right girl. I focused all of my energy and attention on the first goal of going to medical school.

I became a student at The George Washington University. I spent the next three years preparing for medical school. I had stellar grades and my MCAT scores were above average. My extracurricular activities were all geared toward making me look good on the medical school application. I spent two summers as an intern at the National Institutes of Health in the Pathology department's Clinical Chemistry lab doing biomedical research. While there, I was published as an author in two scientific articles in the Journal of Clinical Chemistry. During the school year I was a volunteer at the GW Hospital and I also worked in an on campus research lab as a research assistant. I had demonstrated that I was willing to work hard and get good results.

Yet, at the start of my senior year in August of 1995, I was depressed again. I had applied to 5 different medical schools and had not heard back from any of them. Most of my friends had already been on several interviews and some of them had received their letters of acceptance. I did have one glimmer of hope. University of Kentucky asked me to go for an interview but it turned out that they had already filled their class and they were interviewing for their waitlist. The interviewer at UK asked me how I was going to pay for medical school. I stuttered and stumbled over my words and when I was done, I had told him that I would be using financial aid and student loans. I should have told him about my imaginary rich uncle. Needless to say, they did not accept me into med school.

The realization that medical school wasn't going to happen was such a harsh and devastating reality that I decided to drop out of college. I decided that I had just wasted the last 3 years of my life focusing on this dream of becoming a doctor. I felt completely worthless, so I quit.

I stopped going to my classes and started drinking. One of my roommates, Jason, was a heavy drinker. Jason and I would go out in the evening and stay out all night dinking. We would return home to our dorm in the morning, sleep all day, and begin again the next evening. I did that every night for the next two months.

One evening, Jason and I walked into the bar and within 10 minutes we had already racked up a $90 tab. Then Jason threw back the next shot and as he slammed the shot glass on the bar counter, he said "A real man can hold his liquor." I don't know if he was quoting a movie line or if that's what he truly believed. Regardless of why he said it, the statement felt like a bucket of ice water poured over my head. My image of a "real man" was very different. A real man doesn't have trouble standing tall or walking straight. A real man doesn't slur his speech and certainly a real man doesn't puke in public. A real man doesn't walk away from his dream and a real man doesn't run away from responsibility. Yet those were all things I was doing. Now, I was done. I pulled money out of my pocket and threw it on the counter. Then without saying a word I walked out of the bar and walked back to campus housing.

I was embarrassed and ashamed. I was throwing it all away just because things hadn't turned out exactly as planned. I had a job offer from the National Institutes of

# The StressProof Life

Health to continue biomedical research and I would be getting a degree from The George Washington University, and I would still have the opportunity to apply to Medical school the next year. However, all of that would disappear if I dropped out of school or failed to graduate. I felt so extremely stupid for the way I had behaved. How was I going to crawl out of this mess?

I lied down on my bed in my dorm room and began to pray. I asked God's forgiveness and then, I asked Him to help me get back on track. I planned to start attending my classes and meet with my professors to discuss how I could catch up. I knew that this would be nearly impossible. I was a senior chemistry major. My classes were Physical Chemistry, Advanced Experimental Organic Chemistry, Instrumental Analytical Chemistry, and Inorganic Chemistry. I also had a couple of sociology classes. When I was a freshman, we would have over a hundred people in some of my classes but in these senior-level courses, we only had between 5 and 15 students in each class. I was going to stick out like a sore thumb returning to class after being absent for two months.

The first class I attended the next day was my Physical Chemistry class taught by Dr. Petrina Georgopoulos, professor of chemistry. She was fairly young and attractive with shoulder length black hair and brown eyes and a slim athletic build. She had a very dry sense of humor and very little sympathy for my situation. "I don't think you can pass the final," she said in her Greek accent, "but if you do, that will be your final grade for the semester." I thought that went well. Next would be Dr. Majeed Alhousein, professor of my Instrumental Analytical Chemistry class.

"Absolutely not," he said in his deep and forceful tone of voice. He was a short and chubby man with black hair around his head, bald on top and had a very thick black mustache. It took a lot of begging and pleading to change his mind but he finally did agree to allow me to sit for the final exam. My other professors followed suit.

Sitting in those classrooms was pointless because I was so far behind on my understanding of the subject matter that it might as well have been a foreign language that the professors were speaking. I decided that my time would be better spent at home with my textbooks. I would have to start at the beginning. So I packed my belongings and moved out of the dorms and back home to my mother's house which was only thirty minutes away. I figured mom would be a better roommate for me than Jason at that time.

At home, I would get out of bed at 6:00 in the morning and study continuously until 2:00 in the morning. Then I would sleep for four hours and begin again. I sat and studied at the same dining room table near the wall where the big mirror used to hang.

I opened my Physical Chemistry textbook to page one but just as I started to read, I realized that I wasn't going to get anywhere unless I knew calculus. Well, I hadn't looked at a calculus problem since my freshman year, three years prior. I had to run out and find a calculus textbook and begin my review. This was going to be an uphill battle and one I was likely to lose.

Fast forward to that incredible day on November 25th, 1995, when my entire life would change. That was Black Friday, the day after Thanksgiving. I had been operating on four hours of sleep per night for over a week and I was beyond exhausted. My alarm clock rang at 6:00 a.m. I slowly slid out of bed and even though I was upright, I felt like I was slowly crawling toward the bathroom. As the warm water of the shower started to pour over my head, I felt a strong urge to cry. My final exams were 10 days away and I didn't even have an inkling of confidence that I would be ready for them. So, just as I had done in the past, I began to pray.

I stayed in the shower a bit longer that day and for the first time it felt like I was having a conversation with God and not just a one-sided prayer. I asked God to help me get through this near-impossible situation. I felt like God was telling me that I'm missing something, something important. So I asked Him to tell me what I was missing. "Why do I feel so empty and why do I keep sabotaging myself?"

I suddenly remembered as a young teenager walking into the house to find my mom and Nancy studying the bible. Nancy was a beautiful older lady with short brown hair and always wore a conservative blouse and skirt. She and my mother had met at an Arabic Christian church, which is ironic because no one in my family speaks Arabic. They read together every Wednesday evening. Throughout my high school years and even during the summers when I was home from college, every Wednesday Nancy would ask if I would like to join them and I would politely refuse. I didn't need their bible because I already had a great relationship with God. After all, God had stopped the rain so I could go to the beach, and God had canceled my piano lesson so I could play in the famous soccer game, and God had broken the mirror in the dining room to give me a sign that he loved me and had forgiven me. Why would I need to study the bible? So, I would go upstairs and play videogames in my room. Sometimes, I would hear them downstairs going over a story from the bible and I would just listen because it was interesting, but I never wanted to be a part of the conversation. They talked a lot about Jesus.

"Is that what I'm missing?" I asked God in the shower. "Is that why I feel so helpless and hopeless and empty?" I felt like God answered me. I didn't hear any voices and I didn't see any visions. It wasn't like an angel appeared to me or anything like that. Actually that would've probably made me fly out of the shower and check myself into the nearest mental hospital.

The best way I can explain it is that it felt like I was remembering an old conversation. It seemed as if a memory of a past event was suddenly downloaded into my brain. The memory was of a conversation with God and even though such a conversation had never taken place, it was as if I was remembering a past event. Here's how the conversation went.

"Amir, do you love me?"

"Of course I do."

"Do you know that I love you?"

"For sure."

"What if you had a son, you loved and adored your son and you were really proud of him, but I said to you that I don't really believe that's your son? In fact, assume that I told you I don't have much respect for him. Assume that I said he seems like a pretty good guy but I don't really like him as much as I love you. How would you feel about me?"

"That certainly would ruin our relationship," I thought. "Why would you ask me that?"

No answer.

Then it suddenly hit me. I remembered watching the movie of Jesus when I was very little. I remember that according to the movie, Jesus was the one and only son of God. I then remembered how Nancy and my mother would speak about Jesus with such reverence and respect. "Are you asking me to begin worshiping Jesus?" I asked in an audible whisper. "Is that what I'm missing? Is that why I feel helpless and hopeless and empty?"

Again, there was no answer.

I waited silently for a minute and then I got down on my knees and prayed again. "Lord Jesus, I now acknowledge that you are the son of God, the one who was sent to bear the burden of my sins to die on a cross to pay the price for my mistakes. I accept your gift of salvation and I thank you. I will now declare that you are the risen son of God, and I will follow you for the rest of my life. Amen."

I used to make fun of born-again Christians. Now I was one of them. I had to make sure I hadn't misunderstood and that this really was what God wanted. "God, I need a sign. Just like four years ago when I asked you for a sign and you broke that mirror, I now need another sign. Please give me a sign that is unmistakable and shows me beyond a shadow of a doubt that following Christ is what you want for me." Oh and I almost forgot, "in the name of Jesus, Amen." That part of praying was foreign to me but I thought all Christians ended their prayers like that.

I left the shower and walked downstairs. The house was quiet. I sat down at the dining table and started studying. I noticed that I felt different. I was more relaxed and peaceful and as a result I was able to study better.

Concepts that I normally had to read two or three times to understand now made sense to me on the first attempt. I was beginning to feel hopeful that perhaps I would be able to pass my finals.

I decided that I would stop every hour and pray. So at 50 minutes past the hour I would close the books and bow my head and pray – thanking God for today and the conversation in the shower. I also would ask for wisdom and strength of memory so that I could learn and retain the material I was reading, and that I would eventually pass my final exams.

At around 10:50 in the morning, once again I closed the books for my ten minute prayer break from studying. But for some reason, this time instead of praying I walked into the living room and turned on the TV. The image on the screen slowly brightened and came into focus. I could hardly believe what I was looking at. It was Jesus on our TV. He was carrying the cross that he would be crucified on. Out of sheer exhaustion, Jesus collapsed to the ground. Then Charlton Heston (the guy who played Moses in the Ten Commandments movie) ran over to give him some water. That's when I realized I was watching the movie Ben Hur. I had never seen this movie in its entirety and I had no idea that Jesus had a cameo in it. That must have been the sign that I had asked God for.

I turned off the TV and got down on my knees for the second time that day. I thanked Him for my sign. Just as I had asked, my sign was unmistakable and now I knew beyond a shadow of a doubt that God had invited me to be His child and to follow His son Jesus. It was overwhelming to know that twice I had asked for a sign, and twice God had been humble enough to answer my prayers.

I returned to my studies and continued my routine of studying for 50 minutes and praying for 10 minutes every hour. At around 2:00 in the afternoon, I was just finishing up my prayer when a thought entered my mind. I wondered how it was that we can just call out to God and assume that he hears us. Does God have an answering machine or voicemail that helps him keep track of all the prayers? Or, does He have angels who take messages for Him and only disturb Him if the prayer is really urgent? So, I asked "God, every time I call out to you, do you hear me?"

At that exact moment, the phone rang. It was my mother. "Hi mom, I'm very busy studying for finals," I said failing to hide my irritation for being interrupted.

"Did you eat lunch? Do you need me to bring you anything?"

"No mom, I don't need anything. I'll just grab something from the fridge."

"Well, I'm at Nancy's and we're having a bible study. I will be home in a couple hours."

"You're studying the bible again? It's not even Wednesday. You should have that book memorized by now."

"Yes we are, and Nancy wants to talk to you. In fact that's why I called."

"No mom, I don't have time to talk to Nancy today. I told you, I'm studying for finals. Besides she talks too much. Please don't make me talk to her."

"Hold on, here's Nancy."

"Fine!"

"Amir," Nancy took the phone and began speaking. "I just need to tell you that every time you call out to God, He hears you." Then she hung up the phone.

I was speechless. I couldn't believe what had just happened. I fell to my knees, again, for the third time that day. With tears pouring out of my eyes, I just worshiped Him, praised Him, and thanked Him.

Since that moment I have known that every time we call out to God, He hears us. At this very moment, if I just call Him and say "God," He is right next to me saying "Yes son, what do you need?"

I was hesitant about putting this story in the book. I was hesitant for so many reasons. I didn't want to make public my college drinking days, or the fact that I nearly flunked out of college, or that Jennifer Santiago didn't want to go out with me. At the same time I believe it is important to share with you that the most impactful ingredient in StressProofing my life was my faith. Because, to truly stress-proof my life I needed to put my faith in God and to consider His sacrifice on the cross. The forgiveness, peace, and joy that it provides are unmatched and irreplaceable. To know that the creator of our universe is always there listening when you call out to him is unparalleled by anything else in this world. Loving family relationships, dependable friends, and material abundance, although good, do not come close to the comfort and security that God provides.

So what happened next? I sat for my final exams. I did well on some of them and I did poorly on the others, but in the end, I had passed every exam and managed to graduate with a decent grade point average. I took a year off from academics to work for the Department of Health and Human Services in the Emergency Preparedness Office, and then went on to attend the National University of Health Sciences near Chicago, Illinois to become a chiropractor. If you've read the prologue to this book, you know that a chiropractor saved my dad's life and that inspired me to want to become a chiropractor. Thus came true, my dream of becoming a doctor to help people.

So, what happened to my other life's dream, which was to find and marry the most beautiful woman on earth? Well, that one came true as well. I got the girl of my dreams and together we're raising two amazing little boys. In the same fashion that becoming a doctor had a colorful and somewhat supernatural path, finding my wife was an adventurous journey of its own and the hand of God was obviously the orchestrator of it all. Lessons were learned and the outcome was purely miraculous. But, that's a story that I will save for another day.

What you need to know and remember is that you will face challenges and situations that cause you massive stress, just as I did during my high school and college years, and still do today. If you have faith in God and know that He is loving, generous, and merciful, then you can trust that somehow, something good will come out of it. Through faith in God all things are possible and nothing is impossible. In this you have hope, peace, and confidence that you now possess the armor to withstand any storm. And that is the definition of a StressProof life; not that nothing bad will ever happen but that you will have the ability to get through it, no matter what happens.

# Chapter 8
# *Start a Revolution*

"A revolution is coming – a revolution which will be peaceful if we are wise enough; compassionate if we care enough; successful if we are fortunate enough – but a revolution which is coming whether we will it or not.  We can affect its character; we cannot alter its inevitability."

- Robert F. Kennedy, 1966

# The StressProof Life

When I was 5 years old, I remember sitting in the back seat of my family's blue Datsun. For those of you who don't remember, Datsun was a brand of car that was owned by the Nissan Motor Company. My dad was driving, my mom was sitting in the front passenger seat, and we were headed to my friend's house for his 6th birthday party. I was so excited. All of my friends from kindergarten were going to be there.

Dad was maneuvering through the typical Tehran traffic and we were making good time, until we turned the corner on the street and suddenly came to a complete stop. Protesters were in the street and they had completely blocked traffic. The military police on the other side of the street were wearing riot gear. This didn't look good.

All of a sudden, batons were drawn, tear gas was thrown at the protesters, and fighting broke out. It was like we were on the set of a movie and the director just yelled "action!" Mom and Dad quickly ordered me to get down on the floor of the car and I did. I could hear yelling and screaming from outside the car. Mom and Dad would also utter comments like "oh my gosh," and "oh no!" A couple of times something or someone hit our car and the whole car shook.

I was probably too young to realize the full gravity of the situation, because I wasn't scared. I was just curious. I kept thinking about those action/adventure movies that I loved to watch so much. It was the most exciting thing for me to be in the middle of all that action and I really wanted to look out and see what was going on. So I did. I slowly lifted my head up from the floor of the car and peeked over the edge of the car door. The first thing I saw was a man in a white button-up shirt, gray pants, and black leather shoes walking diagonally toward the rear of our car. He wasn't really walking, he was stumbling. There was a lot of bright red blood on his shirt. He had a full beard and his face showed agony and pain. His arms were outstretched toward the sky as if he was praying. I could hear his voice but I couldn't tell what he was saying. At first I thought I was imagining things but as he took another step closer, I realized what I saw was real. He had a large butcher knife stuck in his chest. He took another step forward and fell to his knees. He then started to fall forward but before his chest hit the ground, I ducked back down to the floor of the car and never looked out again.

I remember that scene today like it was just yesterday. That was the start of the Iranian revolution in 1979. It was violent and bloody. Many people lost their lives for what they believed in. They fought because they believed that their country would be better for it.

I'm not here to discuss the political ramifications of the Iranian revolution. Nor will I discuss my personal beliefs about the situation and circumstance that followed. The reason I share this experience with you is to give you a glimpse into what a revolution looks like. However, not all revolutions need to be violent in nature.

The United States has had its share of revolutions. As a nation, we have faced many challenges. The Declaration of Independence sparked a revolution and marked the beginning of our free nation. What would have happened if the people of that time stood on the sidelines and watched?

The civil war was a revolution. It was a war for freedom of all men and women, and the result was the abolition of slavery. What if people sat around and did nothing?

The Great Depression led to a revolution which produced a new economy and prosperity followed. Those who took action made a difference.

The civil rights movement was a revolution and a fight for equal rights for all races. What if Rosa Parks had moved to the back of the bus? What if Dr. Martin Luther King Jr. had kept his great dream to himself?

Today, America is facing a new challenge. It is called sickness. It is a health crisis and it is killing our people, destroying our families, and crushing our economy. We need a new revolution.

Are we a healthy nation? Look at the numbers. In a report entitled "*National Health Expenditure Projections 2006-2022,*" which was produced by the Centers for Medicare and Medicaid Services in 2013, the cost of healthcare had already reached $2.8 trillion in 2012 and is projected to grow to $3.7 trillion in 2017 and $5 trillion in 2022.[1]
If we are a healthy nation, then why is the cost of healthcare expected to nearly double in 10 years?
Just to put things in perspective, $5 trillion can pay for 200 million mid-size sedan cars. That would mean a brand new car for almost everyone who has a driver's license in America, each and every year.

In spite of all the money being spent, life expectancy is declining. *"Doctors Warned Life Expectancy Could Go Down, And It Did,"* was the title of an article posted on Smithsonian.com on September 21, 2012.[2]

On December 9, 2010, WebMD reported that U.S. life expectancy has declined by a tenth of a year and that this is the third time in the past 30 years that life expectancy has actually decreased.[3]

# The StressProof Life

The reason life expectancy is dropping isn't because the elderly are dying. It's because more children and young people are losing the battle to chronic lifestyle diseases. We need a revolution.

Our children are sicker than ever before, suffering from what were formerly considered adult diseases. Why are teenagers suffering from Type II Diabetes, heart disease, and arthritis? We have made so many advances in medical technology, yet we seem to be going backwards in health. This is not okay. It is not acceptable. We need a revolution.

In the 1980s, experts announced that dietary fat is the reason for heart disease and obesity. You may remember the incredible fat-free rice cake! Following that item, every food company began to produce their own fat-free versions of their products. Thus began the Fat-Free Revolution. What happened to our health? The occurrence of obesity soared into record highs. According to the CDC, "During 1980–2008, obesity rates doubled for adults and tripled for children."[4] Perhaps we shouldn't have eliminated dietary fat.

In the 1990s, we decided that sugar was the culprit. We always believed that eating a lot of sugar and simple carbohydrates could cause diabetes but in the 90's we learned that high levels of sugar in the diet also leads to obesity and heart disease. And because of the removal of fat from our diet in the 80's, more people were eating high levels of "fat-free" carbohydrates. That was why the rates of obesity and heart disease were growing. So, all food companies jumped on the band wagon and began to produce sugar-free products. Thus the Sugar-Free Revolution was born. What happened to our health? The occurrence of diabetes soared into record highs. According to the CDC, "The number of new cases of diabetes changed little from 1980 through 1990, but began increasing in 1992. From 1990 through 2010, the annual number of new cases of diagnosed diabetes almost tripled."[5] That is the exact opposite of the outcome they intended. Not only did it fail to reduce the prevalence of obesity, the introduction of artificial sweeteners, diet drinks, and zero-calorie foods resulted in a threefold increase in the number of people suffering from diabetes. Perhaps sugar-free isn't the answer either.

Today it seems that Americans are revolting against "stress" and calling "stress" the number one cause of disease in America. After decades of adding processed "fat-free" and "sugar-free" foods to the diet, falsely believing that modified food produced in a factory is superior to nature, we are seeing that our health is significantly worse than ever. So, now the so-called experts have turned away from blaming fat and sugar, and are focusing on fighting a new foe called "stress." Stress is deemed the new culprit for poor health.

"Stress doesn't only make us feel awful emotionally, it can also exacerbate just about any health condition you can think of,"[6] says Jay Winner, MD, author of *Take the Stress Out of Your Life* and director of the Stress Management Program for Sansum Clinic in Santa Barbara, California.

So many healthcare trend-setters of today want you to take the stress out of your life. Would you like to know what a stress-free country looks like? It's a country full of couch potatoes. It's a country with high unemployment rates and zero entrepreneurs. It's a country that produces nothing and new inventions are non-existent. That is not what this beautiful nation was created to be by our forefathers. We need a revolution.

All great endeavors come with a degree of stress. Anything worth doing is stressful. Pursuing higher education has stress. Starting a family comes with stress. Building a new business is full of stress. Chasing your dream will be stressful. Living a "stress-free" life means you won't do any of those things.

But, this is America, the Land of Opportunity and the place where dreams come true. Going "stress-free" will be the death of that. It will have the same effect that going "fat-free" and "sugar-free" had on our people. So, don't let it happen. Tell everyone you know that stress is not the problem. The inability to handle stress is the problem. How great our nation becomes depends upon how much stress we as citizens can handle. We need a revolution.

So who do you think should solve this problem? The government's efforts to make drugs and surgery more accessible will help the sick, but it will not answer the question of why so many of our citizens are so deathly ill. The pharmaceutical companies are producing medication that can only help after disease has overtaken the body. The result is more drugs that mask symptoms without any effort toward prevention of disease. The insurance companies have a financial obligation to their stakeholders to protect profits and the only way to do so is by denying necessary services and reducing the doctor's reimbursements. As a result doctors are required to see more patients in less time in order to earn the same amount of income. A good number of doctors are choosing not to participate with insurance companies anymore. Those medical professionals, who proclaim the benefits of early detection, are only concerned about catching diseases earlier and intervening faster. Their efforts are not contributing anything toward prevention and elimination of the cause of disease. The whole system is a house of cards and it's about to collapse on us. We need a revolution.

On the other hand, the chiropractic profession is focused on improving the function of the body in order to make people more resilient against disease. In a discussion post on www.Mercola.com, Dr. Mercola made the following statement: "Additionally, researchers have also found that chiropractic adjustments affect the chemistry of biological processes on a cellular level! And that chiropractic care can affect the basic physiological processes that influence oxidative stress and DNA repair. So there's a whole lot more to chiropractic care than just whipping bones into place."[7]

Dr. Mercola was referring to the famous serum thiol study which stated that patients under long-term chiropractic care demonstrated significantly higher thiol levels in their blood. Serum thiol is used by the cells of the body to protect and repair our DNA, thereby reducing the effects of aging and preventing cancer.[8] By that fact alone, chiropractic should be a staple in every person's lifestyle.

On November 26, 2000, the Chicago Tribune published an article entitled "First Line of Defense, New Respect Boosts Chiropractic as a Mainstream Therapy." Staff writer Connie Lauerman, reported on an HMO insurance company that utilizes chiropractors as the primary care physicians in Illinois. According to the article, replacing the medical doctor with chiropractors as the general practitioners resulted in an almost 80 percent reduction in hospitalization, an almost 85 percent reduction in outpatient surgery, and a 56 percent drop in pharmaceutical drug usage.[9]

These are not small numbers. Statistically, even a 10% reduction in hospitalization, outpatient surgery, and pharmaceutical drug usage would be an astounding savings for the federal budget. What would the economy look like if the cost of healthcare was cut by half? This is not just a money issue. The dollars spent are representative of sick and suffering people. So if hospitalizations are reduced, that means less people in hospitals, less people disabled, less people in nursing homes, and certainly fewer grieving family members. We need a revolution.

In the article "*Medicare Folly*," Dr. Christopher Kent discussed the results of a study that surveyed 311 chiropractic patients aged 65 years or older. The chiropractic patients were compared with US citizens of "similar health status" and same age. The results revealed that the chiropractic patients "spent only 31% of the national average for health care services." He furthermore reported that "the chiropractic patients also experienced 50% fewer medical provider visits compared with US citizens of the same age." In other words when chiropractic was properly utilized, people spent nearly 70% less money on healthcare and needed 50% fewer doctor visits.[10]

There's no question about it. We need a revolution.

In his inaugural address in 1961 president John F. Kennedy said: "Now the trumpet summons us again – not as a call to bear arms, though arms we need – not as a call to battle, though embattled we are – but a call to bear the burden of a long twilight struggle, year in and year out, 'rejoicing in hope; patient in tribulation,' a struggle against the common enemies of man: tyranny, poverty, disease, and war itself.... Will you join in that historic effort?"

Today, if he was alive, President Kennedy may speak the same words about healthcare and ask us to step up to this challenge. We don't need government officials to solve this one. All revolutions begin with only a handful of people, a group of like-minded friends who decide to do things differently and to live life according to their values and beliefs. Let's be the revolution!

All mass movements and social shifts have always occurred because a small group of "rebels" stood up for what they believed was right. Historically, those people would have been ridiculed or worse yet, persecuted, and if that becomes our fate for being healthy, then so be it.

Let's begin by StressProofing our lives. Let's take charge of our health. Let's reclaim our lives. Then, let's set an example for our children and grandchildren and those who look up to us. Let's get our friends and co-workers involved and build StressProof small groups. These will be groups of people who don't shy away from stress, but focus on improving their adaptability to stress, becoming powerfully healthy and successful in the process. These small groups can lead to StressProof communities. They will be communities of people who value God, family, health, and service to others. They will understand the power of innate intelligence, get adjusted regularly, and implement the Simple Seven. Starting this peaceful revolution is as simple as that. Let's be the revolution!

"Be the change you want to see in the world," said Mahatma Gandhi.

"I alone cannot change the world, but I can cast a stone across the waters to create many ripples," said Mother Teresa.

Be the revolution!

I have a vision, that the United States of America will someday be deemed the Wellness Capital of the World. This is still the greatest country on the planet. It has been my home for the past three decades. I'm proud to be a citizen of the Land of the Free, the Home of the Brave, the Defender of Democracy, the Protector of Life, Liberty, and the Pursuit of Happiness for all mankind. "The greatest wealth is health," said Virgil, one of Ancient Rome's greatest poets. Prosperity cannot exist in a society of unhealthy people. Well then life, liberty, and the pursuit of happiness for all must include health.

The time is now. It's up to us. It is up to you and me. Will you be a part of the StressProof Life revolution? If your answer is yes, email me at Revolution@TheStressProofLife.com. Write "I'm in" in the subject line and if you like, tell me how this book has impacted your life. Email me so that I can personally welcome you to the revolution. Your life will never be the same.

With love and appreciation,
Amir

Sources:

1. "National Health Expenditure Projections 2006-2022", Centers for Medicare and Medicaid Services, Office of the Actuary, Table 1, Page 5)

2. http://www.smithsonianmag.com/smart-news/doctors-warned-life-expectancy-could-go-down-and-it-did-45735996/?no-ist)

3.http://www.webmd.com/healthy-aging/news/20101209/us-life-expectancy-down

4. http://www.cdc.gov/chronicdisease/resources/publications/aag/obesity.htm

5. http://www.cdc.gov/diabetes/pubs/pdf/diabetesreportcard.pdf

6. http://www.webmd.com/balance/stress-management/features/10-fixable-stress-related-health-problems

7. http://articles.mercola.com/sites/articles/archive/2007/11/01/new-evidence-supports-the-safety-of-chiropractic-care.aspx

8. Campbell, C.J.; Kent, C.; Banne, A.; Amiri, A.; Pero, R.W. (2005). Surrogate indication of DNA repair in serum after long term chiropractic intervention- A retrospective study. Journal of Vertebral Subluxation Research, pp. 1-5.)

9. First Line Of Defense – New Respect Boosts Chiropractic As A Mainstream Therapy November 26, 2000|By Connie Lauerman, Tribune Staff Writer.  Source: http://articles.chicagotribune.com/2000-11-26/news/0011260479_1_chiropractic-profession-medical-physician-surgery-or-drug-therapy/2

10. http://www.subluxation.com/medicare-folly/